# THE GLP-1 HANDBOOK

# THE GLP-1 HANDBOOK

*Eating Well When Taking Weight Loss Medication*

# IAN MARBER

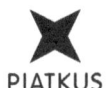
PIATKUS

PIATKUS

First published in Great Britain in 2025 by Piatkus

1 3 5 7 9 10 8 6 4 2

Copyright © Ian Marber, 2025

The moral right of the author has been asserted.

All rights reserved.
No part of this publication may be reproduced, stored in a
retrieval system, or transmitted, in any form or by any means, without
the prior permission in writing of the publisher, nor be otherwise circulated
in any form of binding or cover other than that in which it is published
and without a similar condition including this condition being
imposed on the subsequent purchaser.

Neither the publisher nor the author is engaged in rendering
professional advice or services to the individual reader. The ideas,
plans and suggestions contained in this book are not intended as
a substitute for consulting with your relevant healthcare professional.
All matters regarding your wellbeing require medical supervision.

A CIP catalogue record for this book
is available from the British Library.

ISBN 978-0-349-44695-0

Typeset in Sabon by M Rules
Printed and bound in Great Britain by
Clays Ltd, Elcograf S.p.A.

Papers used by Piatkus are from well-managed forests
and other responsible sources.

Piatkus
An imprint of
Little, Brown Book Group
Carmelite House
50 Victoria Embankment
London EC4Y 0DZ

The authorised representative
in the EEA is
Hachette Ireland
8 Castlecourt Centre
Dublin 15, D15 XTP3, Ireland
(email: info@hbgi.ie)

An Hachette UK Company
www.hachette.co.uk

*For Sue, with fondest love,
without whom . . .*

# Contents

*Foreword by Dr Ellie Cannon*     1

*Introduction*     7

1. What are GLP drugs – and how do they work?     13
2. GLP, weight loss and food noise     33
3. What you might experience when taking weight-loss medication     44
4. Nutrition and calories     53
5. The rewards and risks of weight-loss medications     91
6. Putting it all together     102
7. Your daily menus     117
8. Supplements     141

| | | |
|---|---|---|
| 9 | The importance of exercise | 153 |
| 10 | Looking to the future | 170 |

*Conclusion*     175

*Acknowledgements*     179

*About the author*     181

# Foreword

## Dr Ellie Cannon

This book is essential. It is essential for my patients, but also my colleagues within the medical profession who are now seeing the mainstream use of weight-loss medications and the impact of them, day in and day out – often without any understanding of the profound effects they're going to have on their patients.

The use of GLPs has exploded, ostensibly out of nowhere and everyone suddenly wants to try one. Like a miracle for obesity, it's no surprise they have become ubiquitous very quickly: in every headline, every social conversation and, believe me, every healthcare setting too. And that is because, quite frankly, they are life-changing.

Western society has been struggling for decades with its obesity crisis, which has been fuelled by a food environment of constant grazing and mega-portions alongside a widespread lack of movement. No public health intervention has helped and turning the tide on this modern epidemic has proved grossly unmanageable. For individuals who are overweight, the landscape has been nothing short of grim: constant judgement, expensive fads that promise the world and deliver nothing and the rising threat of serious diseases associated with higher weight. Despite the clear indicators that our obesity issues are national (even global) and societal, the onus and the shame has remained on the individual, wrongly in my view, to sort out their 'lazy' ways and 'make better choices'. In a society that has become obesogenic, this is never going to work.

Time and time again I have rolled my eyes at the latest celebrity or supposed expert claiming obesity can be reversed simply through good diet and exercise; an opinion I heard a writer aptly coin the smugness of thin people.

And then along came the weight loss jabs: Ozempic, Mounjaro, Wegovy. There will be more I'm sure. And they have offered hope and a genuine answer where everything else has failed. An absolute lifeline.

When GLPs work for people – and I have heard success stories from countless patients and friends – the narrative is compelling. I have found it heart-wrenching to see people in mid-life, who were told they were fat at a young age, finally break loose from years of the emotional and physical constraints of obesity. I have had patients tell me that for the first time in their adult lives they are free of food noise, sugar addiction and the strangling cycle of yo-yo dieting. I have met individuals who are in relationships for the first time thanks to weight loss and others who have completely stopped all cholesterol and blood pressure medications.

But life-changing measures come with costs. That is why this book is so vital. No drugs are magic bullets. You shouldn't believe in miracle cures. And that is because all medications, even the humble paracetamol, come with downsides. And, paradoxically, not eating properly, which is exactly the benefit people want from a weight-loss jab, is also a risk of the medication.

Some people don't eat enough and end up tired, hangry, fed up and anaemic when they should be thriving. Some people don't eat well and end up constipated, sick and constantly nauseous when they need to be functioning.

The sudden and often massive shift from overeating to never feeling hunger is such an enormous swing for many people, both psychologically and physically, that it is hard to manage. Many people have never experienced life without constant food noise. So it does need to be managed safely and actively considered.

A lot of people taking jabs have never learned to eat well because of years of being in a cycle of broken food cues and being on a diet or off one with no middle ground. After years of dieting, people often think they understand the good and bad food choices when it comes to weight, but actually know very little about nourishment, what is genuinely healthy and what is important for sustenance. And when you are only eating small quantities every day, you need to know exactly what to eat.

Many people starting a weight-loss jab have spent years in a terrible relationship with food. There hasn't been the space mentally to even learn what really is good food, outside of a weight-loss plan. This is the book to help you now do this properly and healthily.

Consumers and prescribers need more than just a prescription or an online instruction video. You need nutrition advice. If you are going to eat a lot less, you have to eat well and smart so that every mouthful counts and makes you as healthy as possible for your weight-loss journey. This isn't just to lose weight and stay healthy – this is also to make sure you minimise your side effects and are able to keep going. I've come across patients who had to stop weight-loss medications completely, due to side effects which could have been avoided with the right nutrition advice. Some have felt mentally very low on the jabs because they weren't eating enough, or, when they were eating, they weren't enjoying enough of the right mood foods. We often forget this vital relationship between our mental health and our diet.

So far all of the big scientific trials for weight-loss medications have revealed amazing results that keep making headlines: weight loss, long-term health benefits, heart disease prevention and even addiction management. The findings really are surpassing all expectations. But the research also shows that the people who lose the most weight, maintain that weight loss and can keep going on the jabs are the ones who receive nutritional support alongside their injections. We are not talking about this enough: while the medicine itself does the heavy-lifting, a good nutrition programme is a very necessary complement.

Every platform and every doctor issuing weight-loss medication should be offering nutritional advice as part of their package, but, in the main, it is not happening. This is putting consumers at risk of vitamin deficiencies, muscle loss, fatigue and essentially malnutrition. I have already seen this happen because people are not warned how important good nutrition is and what it should look like.

So I will be prescribing this book to my patients on weight-loss injections. Once you've committed to the medicine, you want to do it correctly. And that means understanding the facts and following the right dietary advice offered in Ian's book. You owe it to yourself to do this properly.

# Introduction

I have always had a keen interest in food and health and put this interest on a formal footing in 1996 when I decided to study nutrition. I have now been practising as a nutrition therapist for over twenty-five years. I've been very lucky, enjoying a varied career that has included authoring books and writing for newspapers and magazines, working in media, advising food brands and running a clinic. I have been immersed in the world of nutrition for most of my working life.

I understand and have seen at first hand, innumerable times, how good nutrition can support and enhance our overall health. It can also be used to address specific health issues and goals, such as fertility, bone density, prostate health, menopause, type 2 diabetes, skin, energy, digestion and so on – and this is by no means an exhaustive list.

I have conducted some 26,000 consultations to date, and working with clients remains the central part of my work. While there are a multitude of reasons for clients to seek guidance from a nutrition professional to get the most from the food they eat and the supplements they may take, managing weight issues remains one of the most common – and also one of the most complex. When a client comes to me for weight-loss advice, my job is to guide them through the process so that they can approach their goals in an achievable and practical way that doesn't sacrifice their longer-term health.

When it comes to weight gain and loss, changes rely on an excess or deficit of energy, contained in what we eat and drink, measured in calories. I appreciate that analysing food in such a way can make eating joyless and mundane, but an understanding of this is crucial when it comes to losing weight. However, calories can't always give us the full picture, as they are solely a gauge of energy and make no allowance for the nutritional content of the food. It's the nutrients in food that support all aspects of human health, in the short and long term.

For example, half a small avocado (100 g or so) contains *c.* 160 calories, which is less than 10 per cent of the recommended daily calorie intake for an adult woman, but within that serving we can find fibre, B vitamins, vitamins C, E and K, as well as potassium, manganese and magnesium. Six squares of a popular milk chocolate, or two macaroons from a famous French confectioner, will also contain 160 calories, but when it comes to nutrients there is no comparison: it probably won't come as a surprise that they are minimal in the chocolate and macaroons.

In truth, if weight loss *alone* is the goal, someone can eat 1,200 calories a day of ultra-processed foods and still lose weight. But as well as storing up potential health problems for the future, once the weight loss is achieved and the desire to lose weight is less of a priority, then it's very likely that the weight will return. As a nutrition professional, it's my role to guide clients so that they can achieve weight loss without sacrificing their nutritional needs. After all, there's little value in being slim and unhealthy, having ignored the health implications of a nutrient-poor diet.

But medications that result in weight loss are commonplace these days. At the time of writing The Pharmacist, an online resource for pharmacies in the UK, reports that more than 1.5 million of these prescriptions are issued monthly in the UK alone, and this number is certain to increase as they become more attainable. The most-common medication introduces glucagon-like peptide-1 receptor agonists (GLP-1RA) (there are a few variations), which reduce appetite by altering the way that the human body processes glucose and digests food.

For many people, these are a gift from the heavens. They provide a way to address life-long issues with weight, allowing some users, according to a research project called Surmount-1 published in the *New*

*England Journal of Medicine* in June 2022, to lose some 22 per cent of their starting weight in little over a year, with just one, simple-to-administer, daily or weekly at-home injection.

Although very effective, these powerful medications are not without their side effects. GLP-1 suppresses the appetite, so that eating fewer calories becomes relatively effortless – certainly compared to the cycle of being on and off a diet that has dominated so many people's lives.

The drugs aren't new, and over my years in practice, I have worked with many clients who have taken them. As the newest iterations of the medications, with familiar brand names such as Ozempic, Wegovy and Mounjaro, are increasingly prescribed, I have also seen how they work in the real world. It's interesting to note that Ozempic has become synonymous and shorthand for all weight-loss injections, much like Hoover and Sellotape became synonymous with vacuum cleaners and adhesive tape. I find that clients often use the Ozempic brand name as an umbrella term for all these medications.

My clients tell me how they feel before they take the drugs, how they feel in the early stages and what changes they experience when the dose is increased. I hear about the various side effects, how people deal with them and how long they can last. I will go into more detail about these topics in the coming pages.

## Introduction

But what happens when we don't eat enough? The idea of being underfed might seem far-fetched, but I see and hear of people eating very little. This can take a serious toll on overall health, although some of the effects may not be apparent in the short term. Macronutrients, which is the name given to a type of food, or food groups such as protein or fats, as well as nutrients, play a pivotal role in maintaining a healthy body, but may be sacrificed in the pursuit of easy weight loss.

My role here is offer sound nutritional advice to support the weight-loss plan, ensuring that you still benefit from optimum nutrition when taking weight-loss medication, resulting in a healthy and balanced diet. If you are looking for advice on whether they are a good option for you, then please consult your doctor or appropriate specialist.

In the coming chapters, we will look at how the various types of GLP-1 work, what to expect when you are taking them and how they might affect your life day-to-day, including side effects and reduced appetite. There will be lots of references to GLP-1 agonist medications, a class of drugs that can also be called glucagon-like peptide-1 agonists, GLP-1 receptor agonists, GLP-1 analogues or incretin mimetics. To make life easy I will abbreviate these simply to GLP.

Taking a GLP can be hugely liberating. What has been termed 'food noise' is turned down, so that the desire to eat can be minimised, making eating less far easier than ever before. As a nutrition therapist, I will highlight the relevance of nutrition so that you can benefit from the best that food has to offer – the nutrients that support health both now and in the future – and will also help you deal with some of the ways your body might change. I will show you ways to eat that promote energy, heart health, focus, strong bones, gut health, good skin, sleep ... you get the picture.

Taking a GLP can be a golden opportunity to look beyond calories – and stop focusing simply on whether the food will make us fat or thin – and to change our habits, ensuring that what we eat is packed with nutrients. Doing this when your appetite is curbed can be challenging, and so this book is your guide to how to eat well when you're eating less.

# 1

# What are GLP drugs – and how do they work?

Glucagon-like peptide-1 receptor agonists (GLP-1RA) may well be the impetus behind the most significant shift in the way we eat. Increasing numbers of people losing weight using weight-loss drugs will have a ripple effect on the wider economy, a fact which has taken some businesses by surprise. Yet, had I asked you about Ozempic and other GLPs just seven years ago, the chances are that you wouldn't have heard of them. The hospitality industry reports changes in the way people order food when dining out (two courses instead of three, with more left over), as well as consumers spending less money in fast-food chains and coffee shops. The demand for clothing in smaller sizes seems to have risen too, according to Modern Retail, a

US-based resource for the retail industry; and anecdotal reports suggest that charity shops are getting more donations of larger-sized clothing.

We are offered daily reminders of the phenomena of weight-loss medications through images of slimmed-down celebrities and stories of miraculous weight loss. Share prices in the various pharmaceutical businesses that have developed GLP medications have also soared as their value increases. Closer to home it's fairly likely that someone you know, or at least know of, has taken or is taking a GLP.

I should stress that while I appreciate the life-changing possibilities of GLP drugs, it is not my place to advise anyone either to take them or not; nor to judge anyone who has taken them, wants to or doesn't want to take them. But as someone who has seen the struggle and misery that carrying extra weight can cause, rightly or wrongly, the potential of these medications is nothing short of astounding. It's not all plain sailing, of course, as these are powerful medications and not without risk of unwelcome side effects, some of them serious.

While taking medication for any issue is a private matter, some people are quite open about GLP, whereas others prefer not to share any information about their experience. I'll be looking at this in more detail in the next chapter, but the secrecy around weight-loss medication makes it hard to know the true extent of GLP use in the UK. However, we do know that 1.5 million prescriptions are being written every month. But in the US the numbers are truly astounding. The KFF (The Kaiser Family Foundation), an independent source for health policy research and news, reported that in 2024 some 12 per cent of adults used GLP at some point, with 6 per cent – that's over 15 million adults – currently taking a weight-loss medication.

The speed at which these GLPs have become so popular suggests that the medication is new, but in truth they have been around for a very long time in one form or another. The origins of GLP date all the way back to 1906, when a team of researchers in Liverpool demonstrated that a hormone in the gut could lower levels of glucose (a simple sugar and the primary source of energy for the body) found in the blood. These hormones were called incretins.

From identifying the hormone and incretins to the creation of today's GLP medications, the research and investment has been remarkable. The medications were originally developed to help manage type 2 diabetes, but with continued innovation the latest iterations have been created specifically to combat obesity as they can lead to significant weight loss.

## Glucose – a brief tour

Guiding clients through an understanding of glucose, energy and appetite has always been a fundamental part of my work. The process of creating glucose from what we eat and drink is highly complex. While there is no need here to delve into all of the complexities, I will cover some of the basics so that we can understand how GLP works. This will be especially useful when it comes to looking more closely at how GLP compares to familiar ways of dieting, and how we respond to that in real life.

When we eat, what we consume is broken down in the digestive system, allowing the inherent nutrients to be released and absorbed. As well as nutrients, food is broken down to provide fuel for the body. The primary source of this fuel is called glucose, which is derived mostly from carbohydrates that are digested and broken down into simple sugars. Glucose can also be created in the liver from amino acids, which are found in protein-rich foods.

Glucose is then transported in the bloodstream and delivered to cells where it is used to make energy. But it doesn't just flow unhindered into the cells: it is marshalled in by the hormone insulin, which is made in the pancreas. Like glucose, insulin travels in the blood, and encourages cells to absorb circulating glucose.

Cells can only absorb so much glucose, so any excess is first stored away in a water-based liquid called glycogen, which is found primarily in the muscles and liver. Glycogen acts like short-term storage, and so when there isn't enough circulating glucose, the pancreas will release another hormone called glucagon, which travels to the liver where it triggers the release of the glucose.

We can only store a limited amount of glycogen and when those reserves are full, excess glucose can further be converted into fat and held in the fat cells in a process known as lipogenesis – 'genesis' referring to the formation of something, and 'lipo' referring to fat. By the same token, stored fat be converted back into glucose when there isn't enough to be had from what we eat, and the liver can't make enough to meet energy requirements or, indeed, when glycogen stores are depleted.

When the glucose has been absorbed or stored away, and the amount in the bloodstream starts to drop, various hormones then signal the brain that we need fuel. At the same time, the pancreas produces glucagon that triggers the release of glucose stored in glycogen.

One way I describe this to clients is to think of glucose as what's in your current account, ready for use, while glycogen is what you have tucked away in a deposit account ready to top up the current account as and when it's needed in the short term. Fat stores are your longer or fixed-term deposits – harder to get to, but offering a cushion should the current account and short-term deposit account be running low.

### Glucose – a quick guide

- **Glucose is fuel** Glucose is the primary source of energy for the body's cells.
- **Insulin** When you eat, the pancreas releases insulin, which helps glucose enter cells for energy and facilitates any excess into stores.
- **Glycogen – short-term stores** If your body doesn't need the glucose immediately, it can be stored as glycogen in the liver and muscles.
- **Fat – long-term stores** If glycogen stores are full, the excess glucose is converted into fat and stored in fat cells (adipose tissue).
- **Lipogenesis** The process of converting glucose into fat is called lipogenesis.
- **Fat as energy source** Stored fat provides an alternative energy source when glucose levels are low.
- **Calories and energy** If you consistently consume more calories, or energy from food, than your body needs, you're more likely to store glucose as fat.

## Incretins

This is the name given to gastrointestinal hormones, produced in the stomach and intestines in response to the presence of food. Incretins are produced in response to whatever we eat, but in greater numbers when we are eating a combination of macronutrients.

Two of these incretin hormones are of particular interest in this context: GLP-1 (glucagon-like peptide 1) and GiP (glucose-dependent insulinotropic polypeptide). These play an essential role in managing glucose, and as such understanding how the weight-loss medications work.

Glucagon-like peptide, or GLP-1, works in a number of ways that combine to regulate appetite and promote feelings of fullness:

1. By enhancing the release of insulin from the pancreas, which helps glucose get into the cells to make energy; this in turn reduces the amount of glucose that could otherwise be stored away.
2. Enhances the sensitivity of cells that respond to insulin, so that cells are more likely to accept glucose.
3. Curbs the production of glucagon, another hormone that would otherwise increase blood glucose levels.

4. Slows down the rate of gastric emptying, which is the speed at which food and drink passes through the stomach into the first section of the intestines where nutrient absorption begins.

The other hormone, glucose-dependent insulinotropic polypeptide, or GiP, works in a slightly different way:

   1. By stimulating insulin production, helping bring down glucose levels.
   2. Stimulates the creation of fat cells, potentially adding to fat stores.

Considered alone, GiP can make it harder to regulate glucose levels in a positive way and is found in higher amounts in people living with obesity. Yet for reasons that are still the subject of ongoing research, when GiP is administered with GLP-1, the effect on glucose management and appetite is more pronounced than with GLP-1 alone.

I'll be referring to these as we go along, as they are fundamental to the way the weight-loss jabs work, because the substances the jabs contain mimic the natural activities of these two all-important hormones. In short, the weight-loss drugs allow us to manipulate levels of the hormones which in turn reduces appetite by fine-tuning the whole process of glucose management.

## Appetite

Appetite is regulated by a complex interaction between hormones and nutrients, with glucose, a nutrient, and leptin and ghrelin, both hormones, playing key roles.

It's the ebb and flow of these hormones that result in feelings of hunger and satiety.

**Glucose** The body's main energy source helps suppress appetite: when the amounts in the blood rise after eating, the brain detects this and signals that we are full. Similarly, low glucose will trigger hunger.

**Leptin** This is produced by fat cells and signals that we have had enough to eat, thus suppressing hunger. In some people, including many of those living with obesity, the brain doesn't respond to leptin, a condition known as leptin resistance, and so its effects are reduced.

**Ghrelin** This has the opposite effect to leptin and is produced in the stomach, stimulating appetite, hence it is often called the 'hunger hormone'. Levels rise before eating and then fall again afterwards.

In short, glucose and leptin signal fullness, while ghrelin triggers hunger.

## GLP-1 agonists

After that quick introduction to the basics of glucose and the two all-important hormones, GLP-1 and GiP, let's examine how GLP medications work. It's worth remembering that GLP was originally developed to help treat type 2 diabetes, a chronic condition in which the body does not use insulin effectively (insulin resistance), and/or the pancreas does not produce enough insulin to maintain normal blood glucose levels. This can potentially lead to high concentrations of glucose in the blood, which can in turn increase the risk of kidney and cardiovascular disease, vision impairment and nerve damage.

Hormones exert their influence by attaching themselves to specific receptor sites around the body, and in the case of GLP-1, many of those sites are located around the pancreas, the organ that produces other hormones that regulate the amount of glucose in the blood. There are similar receptor sites elsewhere in the body, including the brain and heart.

You may have heard about some of the other effects of GLP medications, some of which may have been unexpected, or at least not an intended consequence of taking weight-loss drugs. These include people having a reduced desire for alcohol, smoking, shopping or online scrolling. It's been postulated that this may be the result of the GLP hormones attaching themselves to the receptor sites in the brain, similar to those that are found on the pancreas. This seems to influence dopamine, a neurotransmitter that is responsible for pleasure and satisfaction, influencing human behaviours that can drive us to over-eat, shop or drink.

GLP-1 agonists contain a substance called semaglutide which targets those GLP-1 receptors. The earlier versions of weight-loss drugs contained semaglutide, but later ones contain a similar but slightly different substance called tirzepatide that also targets those GLP-1 receptors but, importantly, also mimics the effects of GiP. By tweaking *both* GLP-1 and GiP levels, weight loss is enhanced.

GLP-1 agonist drugs can be administered at home with a little pen onto which you add a tiny needle and then press it into whichever area your doctor has advised is right for you. The medications need to be kept cool when unopened. If delivered by courier rather than collected in person, they are kept cool in transit by standard cooler packs. The pens should be kept in the fridge, albeit once opened they can be kept at room temperature (although the providers and doctors I have spoken to all advise keeping all GLP-1 pens in the fridge anyway).

The process really is remarkably easy, as the needles are very fine and small and even needle-phobic clients report that they get the hang of it almost straight away.

However, the pens have a 'use by' date so do pay close attention to this. Oral medication with a slightly different version of GLP is being introduced, which will afford users the choice between pens or pills.

## What does this mean in real life?

GLP medications work to fine-tune the way that the body handles the glucose that is derived from what we eat and drink. They also suppress the appetite hormones that tell us to eat and reduce the speed at which the stomach empties so that we can feel fuller for longer, which leads to a reduced appetite. The result is that we experience less hunger and, ultimately, eat less.

For a lot of people, eating less without all the complications and stress of traditional dieting can be a liberating experience, but there are potential side effects that are certainly not welcome.

## Side effects

All medications carry the risk of side effects, and some of the unwanted secondary effects of taking a GLP can be pretty unpleasant. These are mostly gastrointestinal, and include nausea, diarrhoea, vomiting, constipation, dyspepsia (also known as indigestion, typified by feelings of discomfort and bloating) and abdominal pain. There can be irritation at the site of injection too. Loss of appetite is also listed as a side effect, which may seem ironic but eating very little can have consequences that go far beyond weight loss, which we will explore in Chapter 4.

You may think that a little indigestion is a small price to pay for the sort of weight loss that is promised, but I am pretty sure you might change your mind if you happened to be one of the people who were adversely affected.

There are also more severe side effects, such as pancreatitis and gastroparesis. When the pancreas becomes inflamed, it can be either acute (severe and sudden) or chronic (long lasting and persistent). Symptoms of pancreatitis include nausea, vomiting, severe pain in the upper abdomen or back, tender abdomen, foul-smelling stools and weight loss.

Nausea is also a common side effect. While everyone's experience will be different, nausea generally passes but, as always, you must let your medical professional know and get more personal advice, especially if it persists. Sipping ginger tea can help reduce feelings of nausea. You can peel a little fresh ginger, mash it up a little with a fork and add it to a teapot with hot water and allow to steep and cool, or put the mashed ginger straight into a mug and add hot water. Peppermint or chamomile tea is a good alternative, but I don't advise peppermint oil supplements in this case as they too can cause nausea.

Gastroparesis is a condition in which the muscles

of the stomach don't work as they should, resulting in slow gastric emptying. Symptoms include bloating, belching, nausea, vomiting and heartburn.

As I mentioned earlier, the medication reduces the rate at which the stomach empties to help reduce appetite and encourage weight loss. There is perhaps a fine line between intentionally slowing down digestion to promote feelings of satiety, and stomach emptying becoming so slow that it causes unpleasant physical symptoms. But how can we tell a passing, mild side effect from a sign that something isn't right? In truth, it's not so easy to tell so it is essential that you speak with your prescriber.

All of these potential side effects serve to underline how powerful these medications can be – but, crucially, that GLP drugs should *never* be taken without the full engagement of a doctor or specialist. And side effects cannot be ignored.

## Accessing GLP medications

I cannot really stress enough that these powerful drugs must be prescribed by a doctor or specialist. It is essential that you stay in close contact with whoever that is to discuss progress, doses and outcomes. Do not go it alone, even if things are going well.

There are several ways that people may access GLP medication but before we get to that, let's look at

## What are GLP drugs – and how do they work?

the most common marker used to assess whether a person's weight is healthy or otherwise: Body Mass Index, or BMI, a calculation of height and weight. BMI has been around for a long time and is the most commonly used measure although it isn't the ideal way of measuring what is a healthy weight, as it doesn't account for the fact that muscle weighs more than fat. Someone muscled could have a high BMI, despite having a more favourable ratio between muscle and fat. Furthermore, BMI doesn't take into account where the fat is stored, as fat accumulations around the abdomen are more strongly linked to cardiovascular disease and type 2 diabetes than when fat is stored elsewhere in the body.

Despite the flaws, it is BMI that is commonly used by medics and online sources when assessing suitability for the medication.

Here's how to assess your own:

1. Measure your weight and record your weight in kilograms (kg).
2. Measure your height and record your height in metres (m).
3. Square your height, i.e. multiply your height in metres by itself.
4. Divide weight by squared height: divide your weight in kilograms by the result from Step 3.

For example, if your weight is 70 kg, and height is 1.75 m, you'd first multiply height, 1.75, by 1.75, which is 3.0625.

Next, divide the weight, 70 kg, by 3.0625, the outcome of Step 3.

The result is 22.857

The usual parameters for BMI, as per the NHS, are as follows:

- Below 18.5      Underweight
- 18.5–24.9       Healthy weight
- 25–29.9         Overweight
- 30–39.9         Obese
- 40 and above    Severely obese

However, there are some differences and the ranges vary for people from an Asian, Chinese, Middle Eastern, Black-African or African-Caribbean family background, as follows.

- 23–27.4         Overweight
- 27.5 or above   Obese

## NHS

At the time of writing, GLP medications are available on the NHS for obesity or type 2 diabetes.

The National Institute for Health and Care

Excellence, known as NICE, recommends GLP for adults with a BMI between 30 and 34.9, if they have at least one weight-related condition, such as high blood pressure or sleep apnoea, and if other weight-loss methods have not worked.

These guidelines may vary depending on the type of GLP medication being considered, as well as the individual's medical history.

For type 2 diabetes, they may be prescribed if other drugs such as metformin are unsuitable or ineffective, particularly if weight loss would be beneficial.

Typically, a patient may be referred to a specialist weight-management service within the NHS. Supplies of the medications can be – but are not always – limited and inconsistent, and patients may face long waiting lists.

## Specialist clinics

Some hospital-based or independent obesity and endocrinology specialists offer GLP treatment. Other specialists may also prescribe the medications, such as cardiologists, who assess that weight loss will alleviate risk of cardiovascular disease. A referral is often needed, though some private specialists may allow self-referral. However, patients must typically meet NICE eligibility (see above), with a BMI over 30 with comorbidities, or over 35 without.

Specialists may perform a full medical assessment,

blood tests and lifestyle evaluations. These clinics can often, but not always, access newer GLP medication such as tirzepatide, which works on GLP-1 and GiP, sooner than some GPs. They may also offer combination treatments including behavioural support. These clinics are usually private and so expect to pay for consultations and medications (although some clinics are NHS-funded).

### Private doctors

Private GPs or weight-loss clinics increasingly prescribe GLP drugs and eligibility varies slightly from practice to practice but generally follows BMI thresholds of 27–30 for those with health risks, or over 30 without.

The process usually involves a questionnaire, consultation (online or in person) and health checks which include weight, but also may include fasting and average glucose levels plus blood pressure. These tests can be expensive but are necessary. Medications can also be pricey, and some practices charge a prescription or monthly fee for ongoing monitoring and support.

### Online pharmacies

There are many online pharmacies that are licensed to provide GLP medications, including some very well-known high-street chemists. Typically, a new patient will complete a detailed health questionnaire, and in some cases be asked to upload photos proving weight or recent blood results. A clinician then reviews all the data and, if approved, issues a prescription. Criteria often include a BMI of over 30 but can be reduced to over 27 if the patient has other health issues, such as sleep apnoea or raised cholesterol.

Prices can vary but can be as high as £350 per month, and consultations are inevitably less personal than seeing the provider in person. This route is popular for its speed and convenience, although it does rely on the patient being open and honest about their situation, and the onus can fall on the patient to maintain contact with the online pharmacy in a way that goes beyond just re-ordering the medication. This does also enable patients to manipulate the system to access the drugs when they wouldn't usually meet the criteria.

I am often questioned by clients who wish to continue with their treatment but are concerned that their BMI has fallen below the level they needed to be at to get the medication in the first place.

This is another area where in-person consultations and regular monitoring and contact with the right healthcare professional has the edge. The client can be advised on options, which may include changing the dose or frequency of administering the drugs.

Online pharmacies generally allow continued

supplies, but it can be hard to then switch to another provider, meaning some people are locked in and committed to whatever price they are paying, even if alternatives are cheaper.

I do know from clients that keeping the supply of the medication consistent is a source of anxiety at any stage of the process, which emphasises yet again how important it is to work with the appropriate medical professional to access the drugs.

I have worked with enough clients over the years to know the desperation and misery that result from weight struggles, so I can see how someone might manipulate the system to obtain what they hope is the solution to their seemingly endless battle with weight. But creating a system that allows for such a loophole is irresponsible and suggests that some suppliers are prioritising financial gain. There is a lot of a money to be made from weight-loss injections, and pharmaceutical companies that have invested in researching and developing the medications have become supremely valuable.

With all this in mind, I urge anyone considering taking a GLP to work with a responsible doctor at every stage of the process and keep them informed of any side effects. If this is not an option for you, please still seek medical advice. Don't risk long-term health issues for the promise of weight loss.

# 2

# GLP, weight loss and food noise

Now that you know more about how GLP-1 agonists impact the way the body handles glucose and their effect on the digestive process, let's turn our attention to how someone might think and feel when taking them. Having worked extensively with clients to tackle weight loss, I know more than a little about the world of dieting – not just the nuts and bolts of it but also how people can feel about food and diets.

We all know what a hard time some people give themselves about their bodies and their weight. How angry they can be at what they see as their failure to conform to a particular body size, and for just not feeling that their body is right. I could fill pages and pages with stories from clients about their struggle with food, and how their battle with weight has dominated their lives.

I have a modicum of personal experience here too, because I have managed my weight for as long as I can remember, through diet and exercise, and have been going to a gym for most of my adult life. I realised sometime in my late twenties that I could gain weight quite easily. I also found that the weight came off (not quite as easily ... ) and so kept myself in line, so to speak.

Until a few years ago I had never felt the need to own scales, because I was aware of my weight by how my clothes fitted. That's not to say that I didn't have a rough idea of the numbers, but I rarely weighed myself. There were times when I was at the upper limit of what I was comfortable with (and past that limit too, if I'm honest), but for the most part my weight was stable.

I have at times been modest with what I eat, at other times not at all. I have been cross with myself, frustrated that I have eaten too much, promised that I will cut back sometime very soon and then become annoyed by my inaction. I have over-indulged and then responded by denying myself – ultimately getting irritated with myself on both counts.

However, within all that and over many years, I was able to manage my weight quite successfully. Until lockdown. The Covid years coincided with a lot of personal stress, and I allowed myself to gain weight, without my usual checks and balances. I was fully aware of what was going on (and even when I pretended to myself that

I wasn't uncomfortable, I still had to face up to the fact that I had actually gained 10 kg).

Of course I know how very challenging weight loss can be, and how frustrating it can be to deal with the constant hunger, hoping that willpower will be enough to carry us through the process. I also know that I am very lucky in that my body responded and I lost weight over the ensuing two years. Coincidentally, over the same period, Ozempic and other GLP drugs became more widely used, and so some people assumed that my weight loss was down to that. But I didn't take one, not least because my BMI wouldn't have made me eligible.

When I have been asked about my weight loss, which has been quite often, my flippant reply has been, 'I ate less and exercised, but don't tell anyone – it'll never catch on.' But that really is how I lost weight, getting back to the lower end of my comfort zone. I am grateful that it worked for me, because that's not always the case. If things had turned out differently, I would have had no hesitation in seeing my GP to request the medication.

What has been interesting is that the question of whether or not I was taking a weight-loss drug was most often framed with more than a hint of an accusation, with some judgement in there too. Which begs the question: if people can lose weight without medication, is taking a GLP 'cheating'? And, if so, does that matter?

After all, what's wrong with taking a medication? There are dietary measures one can take to reduce cholesterol levels, but sometimes taking a statin, the medication that can help reduce total cholesterol levels to a point where risk of cardiovascular disease is lowered, is more efficient, gives consistent results and doesn't require the individual to be ever-vigilant. I can't imagine anyone suggesting that taking a statin is 'cheating'. The same could be said about raised blood pressure and hypertension medications.

Some of my peers in the world of wellness are scathing about the power of what they term 'big pharma', but just imagine for a moment a world without the medications we take for granted now. From antibiotics to statins, aspirin to anti-inflammatories, lives have been saved, and countless numbers of people have been liberated from diseases that would otherwise hinder the way they want to live.

Perhaps any discomfort around a GLP medication for weight loss arises from the fact that it is a fairly recent innovation, and maybe that will pass. But why might taking a medication be a source of shame, and where does this stem from?

Let's take a look at how GLP medications fit in with how we think and speak about food and diets.

## Diets and GLP

I have many clients who take GLP medications, and I stay in close contact with them for the duration of the process. I have heard their stories about weight and their feelings around food and diets, both before and while taking GLP drugs.

I wanted to hear as many stories as I could, so I put a call out on Instagram asking if anyone who had taken or was taking a GLP medication would be willing to have a short chat about their experience. I posted on a Sunday morning and by early evening I had received 454 messages from people offering to share their story.

It took many days to work through all the messages and over the ensuing week I spoke to forty people who were kind enough to give me their time. Another fifty-eight generously shared their stories by email or direct message.

I prepared a few questions for everyone that I spoke to, and those I wasn't able to speak to directly sent in their answers to the same questions online. With their permission, I have included their words and relevant experiences in this and other chapters, anonymising their contributions. Although I engaged with a small sample of people, I found that there were many similar experiences reported and so I feel that it's relevant to share these stories.

So, what did I ask?

One of my questions was whether they were generally open about sharing that they were taking medication to lose weight, perhaps because they felt discomfort or shame for taking weight-loss medications. A few people were happy to talk about their experience with friends, family and other social groups, including sharing their experiences online, but most people had only told a handful of those people closest to them.

Some people said that taking medication for weight loss felt like cheating, as they felt like they should have been able to manage their weight without resorting to medication. This was a common theme both for those who had struggled with their weight for most of their lives, as well as those who had gained weight due to other medication or hormonal changes.

I had other questions, the answers to which will come in later chapters – but there was one question to which nearly everyone gave the same repsonse. I asked each individual whether they related to the phrase 'food noise', and, if so, had their relationship with food changed since starting medication.

The answer was a firm 'yes' on both counts.

## Food noise

You may already be familiar with the term 'food noise'; indeed several of the generous people I spoke to were already aware of the phrase. However, a sizeable number weren't previously familiar with it, yet the words still immediately made sense to them. Our body expresses its need for fuel and nourishment through hunger, fatigue, low blood glucose and so on, but food noise is something different – it's the constant internal chatter and thoughts about food and eating, and for some people the dialogue can be loud and intrusive.

For someone who struggles with weight and eating, food noise can be damaging, as it leads to unwelcome negative thinking. In a cycle of indulgence and abstinence, being 'naughty' and being 'good', seeing food as the enemy and as a friend, a source of discomfort and solace, food noise can meddlesome and invasive.

The notion of food noise is not new, although when I work with food manufacturers, the term 'food cues' is used to describe the many influences that encourage us to eat. And there are lots of them.

Take a moment and think about how often food appears in your daily life. I'm not just referring to when you are preparing, ordering or eating food, but also how often you might come across any references to food and eating during the day.

There'll be adverts on radio and television, social media, billboards and public transport. Not just for food, but for food delivery services and supermarkets, recipe books, restaurants and coffee shops, pubs, wine merchants and alcohol brands. Podcasts, television and radio shows might be sponsored by food companies in one form or another. The shows themselves can be about baking or cooking, and now there are even celebrity versions too, pulling in an even wider pool of viewers.

Annual notable events, for example religious celebrations – think Christmas, Easter, Passover, Eid and Pongal – are associated with food, as are major sporting events. For example, if I ask you which food is associated with tennis, you'll know it's strawberries and cream. And who hasn't been encouraged to celebrate a big match on TV with a takeaway and drinks? Even the weather has links to food (barbecues in summer, cosy 'warming' food like soups and roasts in winter).

Making plans with friends and family might involve meeting for something to eat, while social media is filled with images of what and where your friends are eating. And then there's shopping for food. For some people this can be an unpleasant experience, trying to focus on what they feel they *ought* to be eating when surrounded by so many other temptations, as the food noise gets louder. Food really is everywhere, and part of almost every aspect of life.

Rather than that roller coaster of feeling compelled to eat and plan, and avoid and shop, and be good and be bad, finding something like GLP that reduces your appetite and quietens the food noise can feel like the solution that you've always been looking for. But it's not just food, eating and weight that can change when taking a GLP-1 agonist. There are some unexpected outcomes too, which we will explore in the next chapter.

If the phrase 'food noise' resonates with you, then you are very much not alone. Here are just a few of the responses I received:

*I used to think about food from the moment I woke up to when I went to sleep. If I ate well in a day I would be pleased with myself and feel good about my life, but one slip-up and the opposite would happen. I used to plan what I ate and where I went so that I could stick to whatever plan I was on. I lived with food noise for so long but didn't know it was a thing until the noise dialled down once the injections started working. It's there, but it's quieter now and doesn't control me. It doesn't run my life any more.*

Female, 52

*I worked in kitchens all my life, and so it was normal to think about food all day. I was always a little tubby, but as a bloke it was just laughed off. When I wasn't cooking food I was trying not to eat it. I'd exercise all the hours I could find to manage my weight and tried every diet and fad that came my way. A routine blood test showed high cholesterol and triglycerides, and I was sent to see a specialist who listened to my story and prescribed Wegovy.*

*I was worried that taking it would mean I wouldn't be interested so much in food and thus my career, so I was reluctant. But what happened was quite the opposite as I stopped obsessing about food and realised I hadn't enjoyed what I was eating for years. But now I love what I do and what I eat, and I feel I can choose to eat from a place of comfort, as I'm not driven by urges any more. I had never heard of food noise until you asked me about it, but now it makes sense.*

Male, 44

I'm fifty-two and have struggled with my weight as an emotional eater. Food noise is definitely a thing with me. I started on medication and lost around 6 kg easily, but the side effects were horrible – constipation, nausea and acid reflux. So, I stopped. The weight came back, and the food noise started up again, but this time I was more aware of it.

*I switched to a different medication, at a lower dose and it's been like a miracle – no side effects and easy weight loss.*

*The food noise is there, but its manageable now. If someone hasn't lived with it then they would probably think I was being ridiculous, but lucky them for not having to battle daily demons.*

Male, 52

*I have always been active, and my weight has been quite stable. After my first son was born I lost the baby weight quite easily, but after my second son it wouldn't shift. I was still active but despite my best efforts over two years nothing worked. I started on Ozempic after a conversation with my GP, and it just reset me. I have never been a foodie, nor had I worried about my weight before, and so the whole process has been easy.*

Female, 33

# 3

# What you might experience when taking weight-loss medication

The truth is that all diets work, if you define 'work' as just weight loss. As long as there is a calorie deficit then weight loss will almost always follow. Any way of eating that cuts energy intake will do, be that through guidance from a weight-loss club, opting for high-protein choices, sticking to meal plans, ordering deliveries of specifically formulated meals or only eating anything that starts with the letter L while facing south-south-east (I made that last one up, but I bet it would work because it introduces rules that likely reduce food consumption).

When we first cut our calories (be that via high-protein choices or by facing south-south-east), the initial loss in weight, on the scales at least, is likely to be largely water, not least because glycogen (which is where glucose is stored in the short term) is released to meet energy demands. It's held in the liver and muscles in a hydrated form, i.e. with water, at a ratio of 1:3 or 1:4 glucose to water; so for every gram of glucose that is made available, three or four grams of water is available too. So, by tapping into our short-term energy stores, we are more likely to pee more to get rid of the excess water. If you have ever been on a diet you'll be familiar with the extra trips to the loo in the first few days.

As we know, fat that is tucked away in longer-term storage isn't so easily accessible, and in broad terms, one would need to have a calorie deficit of anywhere between roughly 500 and 750 calories per day to lead to weight loss of 0.5–1kg (1–2lb), a week, at least for the first few months.

It's generally agreed by medical professionals that this level of weight loss is safe, sensible and appropriate. It reflects the rate at which fat cells realistically release their stores to provide energy to cover the shortfall created through diet and exercise.

After being in a prolonged calorie deficit, weight loss is likely to slow. This is because our metabolic rate, which refers to the amount of energy we use in a given time period, adapts. On top of the calorie deficit created by eating less, adding in increased physical activity creates an extra energy deficit that effectively further forces the body to access its stores of energy to make up the shortfall.

All of this requires human input, as we have to eat in a certain way consistently – and adhering to the diet might mean hunger, cravings, frustration ... If you have ever been on a diet you'll know all about how challenging it can be to stick to one, day in and day out, while also somehow making it work despite the realities of day-to-day life. Social events, having a bad day, being short of time, or simply being hungry and fancying a treat can all lead to falling off the wagon. And what about exercise? If you have been able to incorporate increased physical activity into your routine, what happens if you can't be consistent for a while, perhaps because of lack of time, bad weather or an injury? It's harder to keep up the positive eating when things aren't going to plan.

However, GLP medications have changed everything. As we know, they suppress the appetite through blood glucose control and the slowing of the digestive process, which makes it much easier for us to eat less and to maintain a calorie deficit. The outcome is that weight loss is likely to be greater than the 0.5–1kg a week that we were previously used to, and this extra weight can be lost without feeling like we need to do much.

Effective, easy and rapid weight loss is a good thing, isn't it? Well, yes, but we need to be aware that not all the weight loss is down to fat being broken down to meet energy requirements. Along with the fat loss, there's loss of muscle too.

And this is one of the most common and worrying side effects I see in my clinic when working with clients taking GLP medication. It may not seem like an immediate side effect in the way that, say, nausea or constipation might be, but to my mind it's a big deal and has the potential to contribute to long-term health issues in the future.

## Muscle loss

Muscles aren't just the obvious visible ones that can be worked on to increase in size, perhaps for aesthetic reasons. Muscle tissue is found throughout the human body and constitutes some 40 per cent of the weight of the body, although that can vary according to sex (men can have slightly more than women). In addition, the amount of muscle we have can be influenced by age, activity and also nutritional health.

But what is muscle, and what roles do muscles perform?

- Muscle is soft tissue that is located throughout the body.
- There are three types: skeletal muscle, smooth muscle and cardiac muscle.

- Muscles are made of fibres consisting of long cells that interact to cause contraction and relaxation, resulting in movement.
- Muscle also contains blood vessels, connective tissue and lymphatics.
- Muscles move in response to signals from the brain and require energy derived from food.
- The movement can be voluntary or purposeful, such as walking, carrying things, talking, etc. Such movements are under conscious control.
- Muscles are located all over the body, for example in the stomach and intestines and heart (cardiac muscle), and these muscles do their jobs without any conscious input from us.

When weight loss is too rapid and the body needs to access more energy than can be supplied by breaking down fat cells, it will force the muscles to break down too, in order to meet the shortfall.

It's estimated that of the typical weight loss that is achieved when using GLP medication, some 25–39 per cent is actually muscle, not fat. On the scales you'll weigh less for sure, but with muscle loss of that magnitude, there are potential repercussions.

There is a name for age-related muscle loss, 'sarcopenia', which comes from the Greek terms for flesh – *sarx* – and loss – *penia*. This can start in one's forties, gathering pace with time so that by the time we are in our sixties, we might be losing some 8 per cent of overall muscle mass per decade. Sarcopenia can also occur when taking GLP drugs if the weight loss is too rapid, forcing muscles to be mined as a source of fuel to make up the shortfall. This can happen in younger people unless steps are taken to maintain muscle mass.

There are a number of consequences of muscle loss:

- Increased fatigue.
- Increased risk of fractures and falls.
- Reduced insulin sensitivity.
- Reduced immune function.
- Increased risk of chronic disease.

Loss of muscle mass can also affect how GLP medications work. As we saw in Chapter 1, GLP can improve the way that the cells respond to insulin, resulting in glucose flowing more readily into cells to make energy. Yet a loss in muscle mass has the exact opposite effect by reducing the sensitivity of cells to the action of insulin, a situation called insulin resistance, which is itself a barrier to weight loss and is more often linked to type 2 diabetes. When intake of GLP is reduced or stopped, there is every chance that the impaired glucose control will contribute to the amount and speed at which weight is regained. Incidentally, the next generation of GLP medications may have tweaks that help spare muscle loss, but even if they are successful in doing so, they are some way off.

But all is not lost. In the coming chapters I will explain how to manage your weight loss through diet and exercise in a way that promotes muscle maintenance.

## Skin quality and fat loss

Rapid weight loss can also affect the quality and look of skin. With traditional dieting, the speed at which fat cells are emptied is relatively modest, which allows the skin to adapt to the changing shape of the tissue it covers. But rapid weight loss doesn't allow the skin to readjust in the same way, which can result in loose and crêpey skin, giving rise to the disparaging term 'Ozempic face'.

Add in some muscle loss, and the changes in skin can be more apparent; the skin around the muscles is likely to be slow to mould to the reduction in mass. This can be especially evident in areas such as biceps, upper arms, stomach and bum. Just so you can visualise this, it's akin to the loss of elasticity and tone that one might see in a much older person.

And speaking of age, the effect on the skin can be more pronounced in older people who already have a degree of age-related loss of elasticity and reduced levels of collagen.

But as well as muscle maintenance, you'll find there's advice on how to offset skin changes in the coming pages too, which includes not just what to eat, but a couple of supplements that can help as well.

## Changes in other habits

In Chapter 1, I referred to how the GLP-1 agonists occupied receptor sites in the pancreas and elsewhere. This includes receptor sites in the central nervous system, notably in the part of the brain that is linked to reward circuitry and behaviour. This is linked to dopamine, a neurotransmitter that helps regulate mood and emotional responses.

The effects of GLP on other activities linked to dopamine are being studied, but some early research has suggested that GLP could be harnessed to help treat addiction and compulsive behaviours. You'll remember the questions I had for the number of people who offered to share their experiences of taking a GLP. One thing that I asked was if taking a GLP had changed their behaviour in any unpredictable ways.

Some people hadn't experienced any changes, but for those who had there was a general disinterest in alcohol. This applied not only to those who had a drink every now and again, but also for respondents who drank more often.

Research is ongoing, but as long ago as 2013 the use of GLP medications as a novel approach for treatment of alcohol addiction was investigated. In 2021, research shared in the international journal *Frontiers in Behavioural Neuroscience* also points towards the potential use of GLP as a method to treat substance and behavioural addictions, including alcohol, tobacco and various stimulants.

While not in the same category, another change that was reported by my small sample group was that people were spending less time on social media and feeling less driven to doomscroll for extended periods of time. I also heard stories of a reduction in spending and shopping – fewer impulse purchases, if you like.

There seems to be a variety of ways that GLP medications may change behaviours, but what is common to everyone will be that they eat less. In the next chapters I explore what to eat, and show how it is perfectly possible to still eat well while eating less.

# 4

# Nutrition and calories

Whenever there's a conversation about weight-loss drugs, I hear people say, 'Everyone's taking them.' Friends tell me stories of people they know who are on Ozempic or Mounjaro, and the press name celebrities who have completely changed their shape using GLP medication.

Given the criteria, it seems likely that anyone who qualifies for a GLP prescription has already been on a diet and indeed may have a history of diet cycling (losing weight and then regaining it). Some 43 per cent of the adult population of the UK are actively trying to lose weight at any one time. That's over 21 million people – an astounding number – and so a significant number of us will be very familiar with the diet cycle.

There are many reasons why someone might choose to lose weight:

- For a specific occasion such as a family event or upcoming holiday.
- For a medical procedure: some medical procedures, such as IVF, suggest an optimal BMI to increase the chance of a better outcome.
- To cut back after a period of excess over a festival or holiday such as Christmas.
- To combat the effects of medication: weight gain is associated with some medications.
- To lose weight gained due to having restricted movement or limited ability to stay active.

The list is endless ... and there are just as many ways to diet.

There have been countless weight-loss plans, books and clubs over the years – more than I can remember. In such a crowded market, the claims and tailored plans that are being made need to stand out to get attention in order to sell, and this has encouraged whoever is behind a particular diet to suggest that they have a way to lose weight that is a secret, or previously undiscovered, or the favourite method of celebrities or sports professionals.

Each of these approaches might be based around a specific food group such as fibre, protein, all fat, no fat, no carbs or all juice. Some plans are designed to be relatively easy and fuss-free, while others are more complicated and require attention and time. The truth is that whatever the plan, the process is probably all too familiar. You start, you make the changes, you adapt your usual day-to-day life to stick to the guidelines.

And this is because, as I shared earlier, *all* diets work if they involve a way to eat less and move more, as weight loss is dependent on that energy deficit. However they are repackaged and dressed up ... that's a fundamental fact of biochemistry.

That's not to say that some plans will suit a certain individual better than others, for a variety of reasons such as cost, lifestyle and being time-poor. For example, a high-protein diet can be pricey, or unsuitable for someone who is vegan. Similarly, juice-based plans may not work for someone time-poor or who works away from home for long periods of time.

The internal voice – that 'food noise' I described in Chapter 2 – may or may not quieten down. It may do so for a while, but overall success often requires some willpower, as even with a reduced appetite, we stray from food plans. Even with a desire to eat less, there's an element of mastering our desires, as life carries on. I don't think that any diet can match the degree to which GLP medication turns down the volume of the food noise, which can result in not having to rely on willpower – and willpower, as we know, can be limited.

If the plan is overly restrictive or makes it necessary to avoid certain food groups, then in the longer term it might not be practical as life gets in the way. When we're on holiday, travelling for work, at a family celebration and so on, we may not be able to prep our meals in the same way, so it's easy to stray from the plan. Once we have deviated, it can be more of a challenge to adhere to the plan again. Perhaps we do, but maybe we don't. Or we might let up a little and become less rigid with food – after all, we have lost weight and that was our ultimate aim. Once the need to lose weight feels less pressing, it's easy to reward ourselves with the very way of eating that led us to diet in the first place.

The cycle of dieting, easing off, gaining a little weight here and there, getting to a point where we once again feel uncomfortable so that we do it all again, can be joyless and can contribute to poor body image and mental health. The hard truth is that the most effective way to break free of this cycle is to adopt different, more positive habits around food. And anyone who is familiar with being on and off diets will know how much of a challenge this can be.

## An opportunity

I think we all have an idea of what a healthy diet looks like and what foods are generally thought of as good for us. Vegetables, fruits and wholegrains are good, while cakes and biscuits and pizza aren't. Eating well is more nuanced that just 'good' or 'bad', of course, but you get the point.

In the course of my long career, nutrition has become more mainstream, especially as the advent of social media has allowed information to be easily accessible (although not necessarily accurate). This glut of anecdotal advice and opinions has muddied the water so that many well-established and long-understood basics of nutrition can feel unexciting and out of date.

In order to get views and followers, content creators increasingly turn to dramatic and controversial statements to gain traction. We have all seen the 'Five things the weight loss industry doesn't want you to know' or 'Everything you've been told about fibre is a lie' sort of posts, and the attention they attract. They want you to think that health or weight loss is a secret that you have been excluded from, or that it's some sort of conspiracy.

But by pushing the boundaries of what feels like nutrition advice in the name of creating social media content, gaining a larger following and the potential for income, much of the importance of the bedrock of nutrition has been overlooked. Who wants to hear about the importance of dull old fibre when there's a new supplement that will give the best night's sleep, or a weird diet hack that has gone viral?

When I work with clients who are taking a GLP, I stress that their reduced appetite is a golden opportunity to see what they eat through the lens of the nutritional value, not as calories. It can be a bit of a mind-switch, but it's essential to pivot towards considering the quality of the food eaten, not just the quantity. Think more along the lines of: am I getting my 30 g of fibre every day, less than 6 g of salt, and no more than 10 per cent of my daily calories from saturated fat or 30 g free sugars? Plus, all the nutrients at the right level?

Whatever your history with dieting, it's time to have a look at the true value of nutrition and what it can do for you.

## Nutrition basics

In a column that I used to write for a UK national broadsheet, I once shared how I worried that nutrition advice was becoming more concerned about the minutiae, typified by passing trends largely driven by the desire for new content rather than anything truly useful. This was in 2015, around the time of the rise of the superfood, and there were similar discussions and endless copy produced about other foods having their five minutes of fame around the same time, such as goji berries and noni juice.

I am sure all this made enjoyable reading, but the truth is that this sort of interest in novel foods simply served to increase sales rather than make a significant contribution to the nation's health. I mean, it's all very well to concern ourselves with the marginal merits of one exotic food over another if we are getting the basics right – but are we? It's easy to be distracted from the dull fundamentals when people are talking about a berry from the Amazon that indigenous communities have been eating for years.

Whatever your level of knowledge about nutrition, I'd really like you to take some time and remind yourself of the various macronutrients and nutrients, the roles they perform in the body, and their richest food sources.

In the next chapter I will put all this together in some more detail, but, for now, let me guide you through the all-important nutritional foundations that will form the basis of getting your nutrition right.

## The macronutrients

Let's start with macronutrients, which are the nutrients we need in larger quantities.

## Protein

Protein is a macronutrient consisting of amino acids, compounds that come together in various combinations that are used in multiple ways. Found in every cell in the body, proteins are the raw materials the body uses to build and repair tissue. Muscles, organs, enzymes, hormones and even the immune system are all built from the amino acids that combine to make protein. It's the building of muscle and tissue that has made protein a by-word for muscle, and why it seems to form the backbone of the diet of active gym-goers.

There are twenty different amino acids, and the human body can make eleven of them on its own. The other nine are deemed essential, meaning we need to get them from our diet: histidine, isoleucine, leucine, lysine, methionine, phenylalanine, threonine, tryptophan and valine.

Foods that contain all nine essential amino acids – like meat, fish, eggs and dairy – are known as complete proteins. Plant-based sources of protein tend to lack one or more of the essential amino acids, so are often termed incomplete, although there are exceptions. For example, quinoa is a grain that contains all of the essential aminos and is therefore a complete protein while rice, which on the face of it seems similar, doesn't have the full complement and is considered an incomplete protein.

Therefore, getting sufficient complete protein is a potential problem for vegetarians and especially vegans, one that is easily solved by combining foods, as we generally do anyway, so the chances are that the essential aminos will be included (for example, mix rice with some legumes, or top with some seeds, and all the essential aminos will be there).

Protein carries nutrients around the body and supports enzymes and hormones that regulate digestion and metabolism. During periods of stress, illness or injury, our need for protein increases as the body works to heal itself.

If you are looking to introduce more protein into your diet, good sources include:

- Meat and poultry
- Fish and seafood
- Eggs
- Dairy products like yogurt and cheese
- Legumes and pulses
- Nuts and seeds
- Tofu, tempeh and other soy products

For anyone following a vegetarian or vegan diet, a varied intake across the day will generally ensure sufficient amino acid content.

Men and women have different protein requirements, although the general rule of thumb is 0.75 g per kilo of body weight per day. However, those numbers can differ and are hotly debated. But guidelines from the FSA recommend that girls aged eleven to fourteen years have 42 g daily and boys of the same age have 52 g. This increases to around 45 g daily for adult women and 55 g for adult men. In pregnancy, protein requirements increase to around 75 g, which highlights the role of protein in growth and development.

If you are thinking that 55 g of protein doesn't sound like much, remember that the food you eat contains protein, fat, carbohydrates and water too. So, a 100 g chicken breast, often cited as a high-protein food, will contain anywhere from 20 g to 35 g of actual protein. That's quite a wide range, and the variance emphasises the importance of source. In theory a chicken raised in a confined space won't develop much muscle (which is where the amino acid stores are at their most concentrated), but will have increased fat stores instead. However, a free-range chicken with access to a run is going to be more active and therefore the muscle-to-fat ratio is more favourable, hence more protein.

In the same way, an active person requires more protein than someone who is inactive, as we know it helps with muscle repair and strengthening. This is why you'll find many gym-goers and athletes drink protein shakes or take protein supplements, as they deliver concentrated levels of amino acids that help effectively repair exercised muscles, adding to their bulk.

In case you are wondering if you have enough protein in your diet, common signs of insufficient protein intake include fatigue, increased appetite and cravings for sugar, thinning hair, poor muscle tone and vertical ridges on nails.

We know that when taking GLP medications weight loss can be rapid, causing muscle breakdown too, and so it is absolutely crucial for anyone taking GLP to eat enough protein to offset this loss. This has to be combined with the right weight-bearing exercise too, of which more in Chapter 10. As we have seen, muscle loss can have serious and unwelcome repercussions later in life. While you might weigh less and feel slimmer, if this is partly due to muscle wastage, you are not helping your future self very much – if at all.

One more important point about eating protein is that it stimulates GLP-1 production in the gut. This is ironic in a way, as it makes eating protein-rich foods less appealing. It can thus be challenging to eat enough protein, yet doing so is essential to offset one of the undesirable side effects of GLP-1-related weight loss. Another macronutrient, fibre, found in carbohydrates, has a similar effect.

## Protein in foods

| Food | Protein (per 100 g) |
|---|---|
| Tofu | 48 g |
| Soy beans | 36 g |
| Venison | 30 g |
| Pumpkin seeds | 28 g |
| Quinoa | 28 g |
| Peanut butter | 25 g |
| Wild salmon | 25 g |
| Chicken | 24 g |
| Almonds | 21 g |
| Farmed salmon | 21 g |
| Crab | 18 g |
| Eggs | 13 g |
| Cottage cheese | 12 g |
| Oats | 11 g |
| Natural yogurt | 5 g |
| Avocado | 2 g |

## Carbohydrates

Carbohydrates are, in the simplest of terms, molecules of sugars, fibre and starches. They offer an important source of glucose and thus energy for the human body. They have been the subject of a fair amount of debate and demonisation. I am sure we have all seen the popularity of low-carb diets wax and wane over the years.

Carbohydrates are found in a wide range of foods, from fruits and vegetables to grains, legumes, dairy and sugars. As we learned in Chapter 2, once consumed, carbs are broken down into glucose, which either enters the bloodstream for immediate use or is stored in the liver and muscles as glycogen for future use.

Carbs come in two main types: simple and complex. Simple carbohydrates are those that don't contain much fibre, which means that breaking them down in the digestive system is relatively easy and they provide a quick source of energy. Simple carbohydrates are found in many foods that have been processed, even if minimally, as doing so can separate the sugars from the fibre and slow down the digestive process. The processing reduces the fibre content and so allows for the inherent sugars to be absorbed into the body quite rapidly, leading to more pronounced highs and lows in the level of glucose in the blood.

For example, think about eating a carrot – it's crunchy and bulky, and so requires plenty of chewing. The natural sugars in the carrot are bonded to that dense fibre, which requires breaking down, first by chewing and then by exposure to various enzymes and actions as the process of digestion continues. This makes the carrot in its whole form a complex carb.

But put the carrot through a juicer and the fibre

is discarded, freeing up the sugars that were bonded to the physical structure of the carrot. No chewing required. Now you have free sugars, easily absorbed without the hindrance of lengthy digestion. The carrot juice is an example of a simple carbohydrate.

Other sources of simple carbs include sugar, honey and processed grains, but also some milk and milk products. That's not to say any of these foods don't have other worthy benefits, such as calcium and protein in milk, or B vitamins in grains – it's just that they contain easily accessible sugars.

Complex carbohydrates are often termed wholefoods (consider the carrot and carrot juice scenario). You can find complex carbs in oats, brown rice, lentils and beans, and many vegetables.

Fibre is an essential part of complex carbohydrates and plays a vital role in human health. It can help regulate cholesterol levels, contribute to cardiovascular health, and encourage beneficial bacteria in the gut to thrive. It also helps add bulk to the stool, keeping bowel movements regular, which in turn can reduce the risk of bowel cancer.

Consuming fibre-rich foods will naturally help levels of GLP-1, but when taking GLP medication it is still important to be aware of how much fibre you are getting through your diet. The Scientific Advisory Committee on Nutrition report that we consume an average of 18 g of fibre per day, rather than the 30 g our bodies could really benefit from, and so eating less in general risks further diminishing that number. That said, even an increase to nearer 25 g daily can be very beneficial.

As mentioned, we can find fibre in grains, fruits, vegetables, beans (otherwise known as pulses or legumes) and tubers or root vegetables.

## Fibre in foods

| Food | Fibre (per 100g) |
| --- | --- |
| Chickpeas (cooked) | 10.7g |
| Apple (medium) | 4.4g |
| Broccoli (cooked) | 3.3g |
| Baked potato (small, with skin) | 3g |
| Quinoa (cooked) | 2.8g |
| Spinach (cooked) | 2.4g |
| Brown rice (cooked) | 1.8g |
| Carrot (medium) | 1.7g |

## Fats

Fats have many roles and are crucial to health. The brain consists of 60 per cent fat, it forms the basis of hormones and nerve cells, helps absorb fat-soluble vitamins and helps to regulate the immune system and metabolism.

Fats found in food are the densest source of calories with 9 per gram, while protein and carbs contain 4 per gram. As such, avoiding fat in the diet will reduce calorie intake, but then one loses the benefits as well.

There are essentially three types of fat: saturated, unsaturated and trans. Unsaturated fats, particularly monounsaturated and polyunsaturated fats, are especially important. These are found in foods like avocados, olive oil, nuts, seeds and oily fish, and have been linked to cardiovascular health and offsetting inflammation.

You will have heard of omega-3 fatty acids, or simply of omega-3, which are a type of polyunsaturated fat found in oily fish, such as salmon, mackerel and sardines, and are particularly important for brain health, heart function and mood regulation.

Saturated fats found in foods such as butter, cheese, red meat and coconut oil act to insulate organs and can be used as a source of energy, but must be eaten in moderation. When eaten in excess, particularly alongside refined carbs, they may contribute to cardiovascular issues.

Trans fats are either naturally produced and found in modest amounts of many animal products or are produced artificially for use in some processed foods and baked goods. Unlike unsaturated fats, these fats can contribute to inflammation and an increased risk of cardiovascular disease. Trans fats used to be more widely found in food processing and there have been calls to ban them altogether (as they have been in some EU countries), but the food industry greatly reduced their use over a decade ago and there doesn't seem to be an appetite for an outright ban in the UK, in part because their use is so minimal now.

In terms of GLP, consuming fats adds to the overall satisfaction of eating, and slows digestion. By now of course you will know that GLP medications also slow digestion, but fats have many other worthy benefits too.

Good sources of healthy fats include:

- Avocados
- Eggs
- Full-fat yogurt (in moderation)
- Nut butters
- Nuts and seeds
- Oily fish (salmon, sardines, mackerel)
- Olive oil

## Nutrients

Having looked at the food groups, let me now run through the main vitamins and minerals found in our food, with a brief look at what each can do and where you can find them.

## Vitamins

Vitamins are a group of organic substances that are required for all aspects of the body's functioning such as growth, repair and metabolism. For the most part, vitamins cannot be made by the body so they have to be obtained from diet. Some are water-soluble while others are fat-soluble and require some fat for their absorption in the body.

### Vitamin A (Retinol)

Vitamin A is actually a generic term containing several different but related compounds, all fat soluble and collectively known as retinoids. Our bodies can also make vitamin A 'in house' from a group of nutrients called carotenoids, found mainly in red-, yellow- and orange-coloured fruits and vegetables.

**Key roles**
- Supports vision, particularly night vision
- Maintains healthy skin and mucous membranes
- Supports immune function
- Promotes cell growth
- Acts as an antioxidant

**Richest sources**
- Beef liver
- Butternut squash

- Carrots
- Dairy
- Eggs
- Kale
- Oranges
- Poultry
- Red bell peppers
- Sweet potato

The B group of vitamins is a collection of eight water-soluble nutrients that work together to support energy production, brain function and cell metabolism. Each B vitamin has a distinct role, yet they function synergistically with one another. As the B vitamins are water-soluble and not stored in the body, any excess is excreted in urine, with the exception of B12, which is stored in the liver, while limited amounts of B6 are stored in muscle tissue.

Vitamin B1 (Thiamine)

**Key roles**
- Important in the creation of energy
- Supports nerve function and communication
- Helps in muscle contraction
- Plays a role in carbohydrate metabolism
- Involved in making hydrochloric acid so important for digestion

**Richest sources**
- Asparagus
- Brown rice
- Granary bread
- Legumes
- Oats
- Peas
- Pecan nuts
- Pork
- Sunflower seeds
- Whole wheat

Vitamin B2 (Riboflavin)

**Key roles**
- Supports energy production
- Maintains healthy skin and eyes
- Aids in red blood cell production
- Helps support cardiovascular health
- Supports the immune system

**Richest sources**
- Almonds
- Avocado
- Beef liver
- Broccoli
- Dairy
- Eggs

- Fortified cereals
- Lamb
- Mushrooms
- Whole grains

Vitamin B3 (Niacin)

**Key roles**
- Involved in energy production
- Helps blood glucose control
- Maintains healthy skin
- Supports digestive health
- Helps lower cholesterol levels

**Richest sources**
- Beef
- Brown rice
- Chestnut mushrooms
- Chicken breast
- Green peas
- Peanuts
- Salmon
- Tuna
- Turkey
- Whole wheat bread

## Vitamin B5 (Pantothenic Acid)

**Key roles**
- Essential for energy production
- Helps regulate cholesterol
- Required for adrenal response to stress
- Supports wound healing
- Maintains healthy skin

**Richest sources**
- Avocados
- Broccoli
- Chicken liver
- Egg yolks
- Legumes
- Mushrooms
- Salmon
- Sunflower seeds
- Sweet potato
- Whole grains

## Vitamin B6 (Pyridoxine)

**Key roles**
- Involved in amino acid metabolism
- Supports neurotransmitter synthesis
- Aids in haemoglobin production

- Supports immune function
- Helps cell replication and skin

**Richest sources**
- Avocado
- Bananas
- Beef liver
- Brown rice
- Chicken breast
- Chickpeas
- Leeks
- Spinach
- Tuna
- Watermelon

Vitamin B7 (Biotin)

**Key roles**
- Supports metabolism of fats and carbohydrates
- Maintains healthy hair, skin and nails
- Aids in energy production
- Supports nervous system function
- Assists in embryonic growth during pregnancy

**Richest sources**
- Almonds
- Avocado
- Egg yolks

- Hazelnuts
- Mackerel
- Salmon
- Sweet potato
- Swiss chard
- Tofu
- Tomato

Folic Acid (Vitamin B9)

**Key roles**
- Supports DNA synthesis and repair of cells
- Essential for foetal neural tube development
- Aids in red blood cell formation
- Helps regulate new glucose production
- Supports nervous system

**Richest sources**
- Asparagus
- Black beans
- Broccoli
- Brussels sprouts
- Chickpeas
- Cos lettuce
- Kale
- Lentils
- Liver
- Spinach

## Vitamin B12 (Cobalamin)

**Key roles**
- Vital for red blood cell production
- Maintains healthy nerve function
- Helps in DNA synthesis
- Supports energy metabolism
- Encourages healthy sperm formation

**Richest sources**
- Beef
- Chicken
- Eggs
- Liver
- Milk
- Salmon
- Sardines
- Tuna
- Turkey
- Yogurt

## Vitamin C (Ascorbic acid)

Like B vitamins, vitamin C is water soluble and isn't stored in the body, so regular intake through fruit and vegetables is essential. Excess is lost through urine and so we need to ensure adequate vitamin C intake daily.

**Key roles**
- Acts as a powerful antioxidant
- Essential for collagen activity thus skin and tissue health
- Enhances iron absorption from plant foods
- Required for white blood cell activity and immune function
- Aids in wound healing

**Richest sources**
- Broccoli
- Brussels sprouts
- Guavas
- Kiwi
- Oranges
- Peppers
- Plums
- Strawberries
- Sweet potato

## Vitamin D (Calciferol)

A fat-soluble nutrient that requires the presence of fat in the gut for absorption. As well as being found in some foods, vitamin D is made in the skin in response to UV light.

**Key roles**
- Aids calcium absorption for bone health
- Modulates immune function
- Plays a role in mood and brain health
- Helps regulate blood glucose

**Richest source**
- Cod liver oil
- Egg yolks
- Herring
- Mackerel
- Salmon
- Sardines
- Shitake mushrooms
- Soy and tofu
- Swordfish
- Tuna

## Vitamin E (Tocopherol)

Vitamin E is fat soluble and can be stored in the body, mostly in the brain, sex organs, liver and skin.

**Key roles**
- Acts as a key antioxidant, protecting cells from damage
- Supports immune system function
- Helps maintain healthy skin and eyes

- Improves blood viscosity
- May offset inflammation

**Richest sources**
- Almonds
- Avocado
- Hazelnuts
- Mangoes
- Olive oil
- Peanut butter
- Spinach
- Sun-dried tomato
- Sunflower seeds

Vitamin K

Also fat soluble, vitamin K is found in two different forms. One comes from food, the other is made in small quantities by gut bacteria.

**Key roles**
- Crucial for blood clotting to prevent excess bleeding
- Helps maintain bone density
- Supports heart health by reducing arterial plaque
- Promotes bone density
- Supports cognitive function

**Richest sources**
- Broccoli
- Brussels sprouts
- Butternut squash
- Cabbage
- Kale
- Lettuce
- Soy and tofu
- Spinach
- Swiss chard
- Tomato

## Minerals

Minerals, like vitamins, are essential for our wellbeing and our body's healthy functioning. While minerals differ from vitamins in that they can be stored in the body, it's still essential that we're receiving a steady supply from our diet.

### Calcium

Calcium is classified as a 'macro-mineral', a group of minerals that are held in the body in larger amounts; 99 per cent of our calcium is stored in bones and teeth.

**Key roles**
- Builds and maintains strong bones and teeth

- Facilitates muscle contraction to help movement
- Supports nerve transmission for messaging all over the body
- Assists in blood clotting
- Helps release hormones and enzymes

**Richest sources**
- Almonds
- Broccoli
- Dairy
- Figs (dried)
- Kale
- Legumes
- Pak choi
- Parmesan cheese
- Sesame seeds
- Soy and tofu
- Tinned sardines

## Chromium

An example of a trace or micro-mineral as we only need very small amounts of chromium. It is stored in skin, muscles, brain and fat cells, but we need a little from our diet too.

**Key roles**
- Enhances insulin sensitivity which helps blood glucose control

- Supports metabolism of carbohydrates, fats and proteins
- Contributes to cholesterol metabolism
- Supports brain function

**Richest sources**
- Apples
- Bananas
- Beef
- Broccoli
- Garlic
- Grapes
- Onion
- Potatoes
- Turkey
- Whole grains

## Copper

Copper is a trace mineral and we need very small amounts, but it has a wide range of functions.

**Key roles**
- Assists in iron metabolism and energy production
- Supports immune function
- Aids in the formation of red blood cells
- Contributes to brain development
- Acts as an antioxidant

**Richest sources**
- Cashews
- Chestnut mushrooms
- Dark chocolate
- Legumes
- Liver
- Lobster
- Miso
- Mushrooms
- Oysters
- Sunflower seeds

Iodine

Iodine is not derived from metal, like other minerals, but instead is mostly found in sea water and sea vegetables as well as some soils. It's a trace mineral as we only need very small quantities.

**Key roles**
- Essential for thyroid hormone production
- Regulates metabolism
- Supports growth and development
- Maintains energy levels
- Supports brain development during pregnancy and infancy

**Richest sources**
- Cod

- Dairy
- Eggs
- Mussels
- Potatoes
- Salmon
- Seaweed
- Shrimp
- Strawberries
- Tuna

## Iron

Dietary iron is found in two forms: 'heme' iron, which is found only in animal flesh, and 'non-heme' iron found in plants. Heme iron is more efficiently absorbed than non-heme. The presence of vitamin C enhances overall iron absorption from food.

**Key roles**
- Supports oxygen transport in the blood
- Aids in energy production
- Supports immune function
- Contributes to cognitive development

**Richest sources**
- Chickpeas
- Dried apricots
- Lentils
- Liver

- Oysters
- Pumpkin seeds
- Red meat
- Spinach
- Tofu
- Venison

## Magnesium

Magnesium is the most prolific mineral in the body, after calcium. It is a key component of chlorophyll, which helps plants make energy from sunlight, and so is especially rich in plant-based foods.

**Key roles**
- Supports energy production
- Aids in muscle contraction and nerve transmission
- Regulates blood pressure and blood glucose levels
- Essential for maintaining bone density
- Involved in DNA and protein synthesis

**Richest sources**
- Almonds
- Avocado
- Black beans
- Cashews

- Chia seeds
- Dark chocolate
- Pumpkin seeds
- Spinach
- Tofu
- Whole grains

Manganese
Manganese is a trace mineral that is naturally found in soil and sea water, hence it's absorbed by plants and some seafood.

**Key roles**
- Acts as a co-factor in many enzyme systems
- Supports bone formation and connective tissue health
- Plays a role in blood clotting and wound healing
- Functions as an antioxidant
- Assists in carbohydrate and fat metabolism

**Richest sources**
- Black tea
- Brown rice
- Hazelnuts
- Mussels
- Oats
- Pine nuts

- Pineapple
- Spinach
- Sweet potato
- Whole wheat bread

Potassium

Potassium is found in all fruits and vegetables, including legumes, although some is found in dairy food too.

**Key roles**
- Maintains normal fluid and electrolyte balance
- Supports proper nerve function
- Aids in muscle contraction, including the heart
- Helps regulate blood pressure
- Helps energy production from glucose

**Richest sources**
- Avocado
- Bananas
- Cucumber
- Dried apricots
- Greens
- Lentils
- Potatoes (with skin)
- Spinach
- Sweet potato
- Tomato

## Selenium

Selenium is only needed in very small amounts and is found in plants and sea water, hence its concentration in sea vegetables and marine life.

**Key roles**
- Antioxidant activity
- Supports thyroid hormone metabolism
- Plays a role in immune system function
- Contributes to DNA synthesis
- May help reduce inflammation, especially in the skin

**Richest sources**
- Brazil nuts
- Brown rice
- Chicken breast
- Eggs
- Mushrooms
- Oats
- Prawns
- Sardines
- Sunflower seeds
- Tuna

## Zinc

Zinc has a multitude of roles, and while some is stored in the body we need some zinc from our daily diet.

**Key roles**
- Supports immune system function
- Aids in wound healing and skin health
- Involved in cell growth and division
- Essential for normal taste and smell
- Antioxidant activity

**Richest sources**
- Beef
- Chickpeas
- Dairy
- Lentils
- Mushrooms
- Oysters
- Poultry
- Pumpkin seeds
- Quinoa
- Seaweed

# 5

# The rewards and risks of weight-loss medications

You may have heard the somewhat contradictory term 'skinny fat', which refers to an individual who has a healthy BMI (body mass index) but an unfavourable ratio between muscle mass and body fat. When it comes to the numbers on the scales, and fitting into clothes, all may seem well; the person in question may look of average weight, even trim, but have a higher level of visceral fat, which is the fat around the belly and between the organs. It can't be seen, but someone with increased levels of visceral fat may be at a higher risk of insulin resistance. This is when cells don't respond properly to the presence of insulin, and this may in time affect the pancreas, as well as raising cholesterol and blood pressure.

When it comes to GLP, there is another contradiction that may seem a little baffling at first, and that's the risk of being underfed, and malnourished. The confusion here is that while losing weight can help improve overall health by reducing the risk of cardiovascular disease, type 2 diabetes and some forms of cancer, and improve joint health and energy levels, being undernourished carries its own health risks. It's this point that is especially relevant when it comes to getting the best nutrition within a smaller intake of food.

When taking a GLP medication, it's quite possible to undereat simply because of lack of appetite, or indeed to ignore hunger signals because the medication makes it possible to power through on minimal amounts of food.

Clients, friends and respondents have shared their experience of not eating much while taking GLP, and here are a few of their stories to illustrate how this can manifest in real life:

> *For me, the drugs have been life changing. I cannot believe I have finally had to stop fretting about diets. After maybe six months, though, I found I got every cold, I was so tired, I had a few breakouts and was constipated again and again. My nails were brittle and ridged too.*
>
> *I saw a nutritionist and went for some blood*

*tests and found that I had low levels of all sorts of vitamins, which was quite the wake-up call.*

*It's much better now as I understand more about nutrition, but I was shocked to think that I could have gone from being overweight to undernourished in just a few months. I didn't even think it was possible.*

Female, 30

*I couldn't go to the doctor for anything without being told I needed to lose weight. Like I didn't know. Being a size 20 seemed to preclude me from having anything that I needed to see a doctor for without them suggesting that whatever it was would be better if I lost weight.*

*The GLP changed all that, and as my cholesterol and blood pressure came down, I had fewer aches and pains, I slept better, and my mood was better.*

*But I wasn't really eating well. I knew that, but as long as I was losing weight no one seemed to notice. As long as I was slimmer, then I could get away with not eating well because in truth the food I was eating was worse than what I used to eat when I just couldn't be bothered to diet – I was just eating less of it.*

Female, 28

When someone has lived with the effects of excess calories, the possibility of going from eating too much to be being malnourished might seem far-fetched, but it can – and does – happen.

Being underfed and thus malnourished has several implications for health in the medium and long term. There is plenty of research into the effects of malnutrition, but studies investigating the issue as a result of taking weight-loss drugs is scant. However, one cross-sectional study found that in people using GLP, the intake of several essential nutrients was too low. A cross-sectional study is a snapshot, highlighting data in that moment, as opposed to a long-term study. The nutrients that this study tracked were calcium, magnesium, potassium and vitamin D.

So what is malnourishment? The NHS say that one of the symptoms of being malnourished is unintentionally losing 5–10 per cent of your body weight in three to six months. Taking a GLP is clearly intentional, but making the comparison here is relevant, as rapid weight loss has the same outcome.

Over time, it is quite possible for lack of nutrition to contribute to ill health, but as yet we can only make predictions as to what might happen as a direct result of taking GLP medications. It seems obvious that there will be significant crossover, but perhaps there will be some issues that are directly attributable to the way that the medications affect appetite. To my mind, nutrition is the cornerstone of good health, and we can all benefit from what good nutrition can do for us.

We know that there are well-established risks of ill health directly related to being malnourished. These risks are rooted in lack of nutrients, but can be exacerbated both by eating foods that have poor nutrient levels, and by replacing wholefoods with ultra-processed foods. These are foods that have been processed to a degree that they have low-nutrient status, together with additives that prolong shelf life. Even if the foods aren't the worst offenders, then replacing nutrient-dense foods with those rich in refined sugars and saturated fats may further contribute to poor health in time.

Here are some of the conditions that can be directly influenced by inadequate intake of key nutrients. I should stress that poor nutrient intake is one of several factors that can contribute to these conditions.

1. **Cardiovascular disease** Deficiencies in omega-3 fatty acids, magnesium, potassium and certain B vitamins (especially B6, B12 and folate) can increase the risk of raised homocysteine and blood lipids. Diets with limited intake of vegetables, fruits and whole grains may contribute to hypertension and arrhythmias.
2. **Osteoporosis** Linked to low intake of calcium, vitamins D and K, and magnesium.

3. **Anaemia** Low iron intake and absorption can lead to anaemia, poor cognitive function and impaired immunity.
4. **Poor immunity** Deficiencies of vitamins A, C and E, together with selenium and zinc, can lead to a weak immune response, increasing susceptibility of infection.
5. **Digestive disorders** Lack of fibre increases the risk of colon cancer, lack of diversity of gut bacteria, constipation and raised cholesterol.
6. **Neurological issues** Vitamin B12 deficiency is associated with nerve damage and poor memory.
7. **Eyesight problems** Vitamin A deficiency can lead to night blindness, while low intake of zinc and lutein, a carotenoid found in brightly coloured fruits and vegetables, can increase the risk of macular degeneration.
8. **Cognitive status** Long-term low intake of B12, folate, omega-3 and antioxidants may contribute to cognitive decline.
9. **Hair and skin problems** Low intake of protein together with omega-3, biotin, zinc and vitamin C can lead to brittle and dry nails, skin and hair, plus poor wound healing and inflammation.
10. **Reduced fertility** Low nutrient status, especially zinc, folate, vitamin D and iron are associated with reduced fertility and low birth weight.

## The rewards and risks of weight-loss medications

These risks are real, and it is essential to work with your doctor to ensure that your GLP dose is right for you. There's a balance to be struck between the medication being effective, and what is essentially taking a higher dose than is good for you, despite the potential for faster weight loss. You will still lose weight on a modest dose and also avoid being underfed and undernourished.

> *When I turned sixty, I had this realisation that I had been on and off a diet and battling with food since I was a teen. That's almost half a century of not feeling at home in my own body, and while I am used to how I am, it certainly doesn't make me happy. I had worked with a therapist who had helped me see that I used food to blot out issues that I had never faced, and while I didn't have an eating disorder, I certainly had inconsistent and complex behaviours when it came to food.*
>
> *I felt more at peace when I accepted the size that I was, but then I was offered the new weight-loss jab by my GP who had concerns about my blood pressure and joint pain.*
>
> *I started with a very low dose and felt the effects within a week, and it was all gentle and manageable over the next few weeks as I lost weight and gradually increased the dose. When I was at 1.7 mg (the dosage goes up to 2.4 mg) my appetite just*

went. I wanted to eat, but after a few bites I felt full and found it hard to carry on, even though I knew it wasn't right.

The food noise had stopped, but something else had happened as I enjoyed not eating, that feeling of being able to eat almost nothing and feel OK. At one point I was eating no more than a couple of apples and some cheese most days, and then chocolate and crisps at home in the evening, because for once I could open a small packet, have just a handful and that was enough. I didn't feel compelled to eat the whole pack.

I knew it wasn't right, but I loved being in charge of how much I was eating for once. I was losing weight, but I had no energy, and my skin felt dry. I kept putting off telling the doctor as I liked the feeling of not having to eat, but when it was time to increase the dose I came clean. He reduced the dose way down and within a week I felt hungry again, but nicely hungry so I could eat again. Quite soon I saw changes, not just in energy but my skin and nails improved, so did my hair quality.

The idea of being malnourished was so alien, I had never considered it. Food for me has never been about nourishment, only something to be dealt with, like an unwelcome but necessary evil.

The whole experience has changed me, not just

*because I am happier in my body but because I feel differently about food now.*

Female, 63

## Other benefits of GLP

The flip side of any risk is reward, and it seems that above and beyond the impressive benefits that GLP can deliver in terms of weight loss, the medications are delivering benefits in other areas too.

Once again, it is relatively early days, and there aren't many long-term studies, but there are strong indications that the effects of GLP medications may be far-reaching and extend beyond those that result from weight loss alone.

In the LEADER trial, published in 2016 in the *New England Journal of Medicine*, patients with type 2 diabetes at higher risk of cardiovascular disease were given either liraglutide, a GLP agonist, or a placebo. In just under four years, those taking the GLP showed a reduction in what are termed 'cardiovascular events' including stroke, heart attack and fatalities. The trial was funded in part by the National Institutes of Health in the US as well as Novo Nordisk, the manufacturers of liraglutide, but was carried out by some very august researchers from a variety of universities and hospitals all over the world.

GLP is thought to reduce inflammation and its associated conditions. It's common for blood tests to measure CRP, or c-reactive protein, and so it's likely that you've seen this on your own test results. CRP is a protein produced in the liver in response to inflammation, and it seems that many patients taking GLP have a lower score.

Inflammation itself has wide-ranging effects, and so it's logical to see an improvement in cardiovascular disease, some forms of cancer and general age-related decline. Early signs are that this may extend to cognitive decline too, including dementia, Parkinson's disease and Alzheimer's disease.

Inflammation can also manifest itself in the skin and so may benefit conditions such as psoriasis and dermatitis. There is also the potential for GLP to help reduce the severity of various types of arthritis.

All of these ancillary outcomes are very welcome and go beyond what might be expected of the health benefits usually associated with weight loss. When I hear from clients and correspondents they are usually thrilled about the overall results. I work closely with clients to help them avoid malnutrition, explaining to them from the outset that it can be a real concern. I encourage them – and you too – to be aware of changes in appetite. If you are getting to the stage when you are rarely hungry and have little to no appetite, then it is very important to have a frank discussion with your prescribing doctor or specialist. A lack of appetite that leads to even mild malnutrition is not a good outcome.

As we have seen, rapid weight loss can have unwanted repercussions. But in the longer term there is a real risk of health issues that may not be apparent in the early stages. The GLP medications are there to help manage weight in a healthy and positive way, but there is the possibility of misuse, or excess doses.

You may have heard about micro-dosing, where you intentionally take less of the medication either to offset poor appetite or to extend the duration of the prescription (this can be due to the cost of accessing the medication privately). I have seen some advice about the practice on social media, but unless your own doctor, or whoever prescribed the medication, has advised you to do this, then you really mustn't go down this route.

# 6

# Putting it all together

So far we have looked at several aspects of GLP – the positives and the pitfalls – and now it's time to put it all together. In doing so you will be able to see how to eat and nourish yourself, as well as manage weight loss – eating well now that you are eating less.

## What to look for

There is much debate around what constitutes a healthy balanced diet, but in the context of eating when taking GLP, let's start by looking at some well-established guidelines as advised by most health authorities. You may think that all one has to do when eating less under the influence of a GLP is to eat the same proportions as before, but this may not adequately offset the potential unwanted real-life consequences of a greatly reduced appetite.

1. **Fruit and vegetables** These should make up around 40 per cent of what we eat, ideally with at least five portions daily.
2. **Complex carbohydrates** Carbohydrates that are rich in fibre should be included, making up around 38 per cent of our total daily intake.
3. **Protein** This can be animal- or plant-based, including fish twice a week, one of which should be omega-3-rich oily fish. Protein should constitute 12 per cent of our daily intake.
4. **Dairy or alternatives** These should make up around 8 per cent of the intake, favouring lower-fat options.
5. **Oils and fats** These include olive oil, butter and alternatives, making up 1 per cent.

When it comes to foods that we should limit, there are also guidelines to follow.

**Saturated fats** As we know, these are fats found in animal-based foods, butter, cheese and tropical oils such as coconut. In excess, they can contribute to raised cholesterol, which is a significant factor in cardiovascular disease. Our saturated fat intake should be limited to 11 per cent of our daily calorie intake, which equates to 20 g for women and 30 g for men.

Trans fats should be avoided, and are found in some pastries, fried foods, crackers, cakes and spreads. They are often labelled as 'partially hydrogenated fat', which is food industry speak for the process of adding hydrogen ions to vegetable oils. This allows the fats to stay solid at room temperature, but the process also results in trans fats.

**Sugar** The type of sugars that are relevant here are what are termed 'free sugars', which are those that are added to what we eat, either by manufacturers or by us. This also applies to sugars in sweet syrups, like maple or molasses, as well as honey.

Free sugars are also found in fruit and vegetable juices, as the sugars they naturally contain have been separated and freed from the fibre by the process of juicing (think back to the carrot in Chapter 5!). These should be limited to no more than 30 g a day.

**Calories** In terms of calorie consumption, guidance suggests that adult women should aim for around 2,000 calories a day, while men should aim for 2,500 in order to maintain weight, while also allowing for enough food to include essential nutrients that contribute to supporting the human body. These estimates also take into consideration typical physical activity.

Bear in mind, though, that when losing weight there has to be a calorie deficit, so your optimum calorie intake will drop. A general rule of thumb is that in order to lose 1–2 lb/0.5–1 kg a week, there needs to be a calorie deficit of 500–700 calories a day.

I must stress that this is not an exact science, because there are so many variables, such as age, starting weight, general health and level of physical activity.

## How much weight is it safe to lose?

Along with ease, a fast pace of weight loss has long been promoted as desirable. Any number of diet plans and books make the claim that you can lose X amount in a specific time period. This approach is appealing because it promises that the process of a diet won't be too painful or take too long, but any seasoned dieter knows that it's not that easy, and after you come off the diet, you may regain what you lost – and more.

The recommendation to lose weight at the rate of a couple of pounds a week is sensible, because it reduces the risk of any significant lack of nutrients and also allows for fat stores to be broken down to allow energy to be released to make up for the deficit created by reduced food intake. Fat stores can't be accessed all at once, and can be slow to break down, and so losing weight aligned with the way the human body works results in a better outcome.

Modest weight loss allows for this process and so largely spares muscle from being broken down in a hurry to meet a larger deficit than can be dealt with. This is a really important point, because taking GLP can minimise appetite to such an extent that it's easy to create a deficit that cannot be met by energy stores (i.e. fat) and so muscles are cannibalised instead.

Therefore, for an adult woman, one who is moderately active, calorie intake should be reduced from 2,000 to between 1,300 and 1,500 per day. For a moderately active adult male that figure goes from 2,500 to 1,800 to 2,000 calories per day.

By now you will know that taking a GLP can help reduce the appetite to such a level that it's very easy to eat far less than that. Not just easy, but eating that much may actually be a challenge, and so weight loss in excess of 1–2 lb/0.5–1 kg a week is likely.

## Gallstones and rapid weight loss

There is also a slightly increased risk of developing gallstones if weight loss is too rapid. To remind you, the fat in the diet has to be broken down a little so it can be absorbed, and one way that is done is by bile, a liquid made in the liver and stored in the gall bladder. When fat from the diet is in the digestive tract, the gall bladder releases bile to help break it down. You can visualise this by thinking of what happens when you squirt dishwashing liquid into a pan after you have cooked something like a Sunday roast. The bile breaks down the fat into smaller globules, just like the soap breaks up the cooking fat.

Bile is made in part of cholesterol, which can combine with other substances in the gall bladder to form stones. This is all quite normal, but their incidence and number can be increased when losing weight rapidly because the lack of dietary fat can mean, in simple terms, that the contents of the gall bladder get backed up.

Gallstones needn't be too much of a worry if you can keep a close and realistic eye on your appetite and rate of weight loss. Eating enough to fuel and nourish yourself and achieve a modest rate of weight loss should avoid any increased risk.

## My GLP plan

Given all the possible pitfalls, here are the essential elements for fuelling yourself, reducing any muscle wastage and associated loose skin, while still supplying essential nutrients that support and promote how you feel and function.

To be taking GLP you will no doubt have dieted in the past, and whichever your preferred route or method you will have had to be mindful. Whether that meant being aware of counting calories, avoiding carbs, fasting until whatever time and so on, there were rules to follow.

Taking a GLP can be very liberating as it feels like an effortless way to lose weight, almost as if it happens without much input from you. When working with clients who are taking GLP, I always stress that it is crucial that they stay aware of their appetite, and if they find that they can't eat enough, they need to be honest and reach out to their doctor or specialist and discuss how they are feeling – and I encourage you to do the same.

With all this in mind, my plan is based on:

- Calories
- Protein
- Fibre
- Hydration
- Variety

## Calories

*Why?*
To avoid overly rapid weight loss.

*How many?*
On the preceding pages you will have seen what happens when calorie intake is greatly reduced. If energy

*Putting it all together*

intake is cut to a level at which stored fat cannot be realistically broken down to create enough energy to meet the shortfall, then muscle can be broken down instead. Sensible and safe weight loss means a drop to 1,300 to 1,500 calories for women and 1,800 to 2,000 for men. I urge you to get to *at least* the lower figure. You will still lose weight, be able to eat and nourish yourself while enjoying food – without overeating.

A great way to gauge how many calories you are eating is to download an app that will allow you to input what you are eating to calculate your rough calorie intake. Fitness-related apps are often good ones to get, and you only need a free version to be able to keep track. Or you may find that the pre-installed health-related app on your phone offers this feature already.

Rather than enter everything, every single day, do this for a few days until you get used to the process. You'll soon get the hang of it and will be able to judge if you are eating enough.

You may need to repeat the process as your GLP doses increase, as it's easy to eat a little less here and there without noticing you aren't eating enough. Bear in mind too that you may not feel like eating your 'usual' amount of food, and so getting those nutrient-rich calories in is something you will get used to.

In the next chapter I will cover plenty of nutrient-rich meals and snacks. They are easy to make and involve cobbling together familiar foods to create a delicious daily menu that provides flavour and nutrients.

## Protein

*Why?*

I have detailed the role of protein in Chapter 5, but in the context of GLP, it is essential, along with the right exercise and activity, in order to counteract the potential for muscles to be broken down to meet energy demands. Therefore, you need to eat protein and potentially look to supplement with some additional protein (see Chapter 8 on supplements).

Protein intake, calories and the right physical activity can help offset unnecessary muscle loss.

*How much?*

For a woman, aiming for 1.5 g protein per day for every kilo of body weight will be ideal. A man should aim for more, a shade under 2 g per kilo of body weight per day.

*How often?*

Ideally, every time you eat there will be some protein in the mix. A useful way to remember to eat a little with every meal is to always ask yourself 'Where's my protein?' when you are prepping or cooking your food.

## Fibre

*Why?*

Fibre is an essential part of a positive and healthy diet, all of which stands true in the context of a GLP plan. But taking GLP can slow gastric emptying, leading to potential constipation, which is more than just not being able to go to the loo so easily, but can also raise the risk of haemorrhoids, fissures and diverticulitis.

Fibre is found in fruits, vegetables and grains, and so getting a minimum of 25 g fibre a day – ideally more – will also provide a multitude of vitamins, minerals, antioxidants, carotenoids, organosulphides and glucosinolates. Fresh produce contributes to overall hydration too.

## Hydration

*Why?*

Fluid intake is often almost an afterthought when weight loss is discussed, but it takes on added importance when using GLP medication. The side effects of the medication, such as nausea and constipation, can be offset to some extent by adequate hydration. Skin can also be drier and less supple when dehydrated. In addition, when appetite is reduced it is inevitable that we will consume fewer fluids, as we are eliminating the fluids found naturally in the food we eat.

Hydration also plays an integral role in a process called lipolysis in which the stored fats are broken down to release energy. This is especially relevant when taking GLP because we want that process to be efficient as it may help in reducing muscle breakdown.

*How much?*

Hydration comes from all liquids, not just water. You can get an idea of your levels of hydration by checking the colour of your urine. A pale yellow suggests adequate hydration, dark yellow suggests some dehydration.

I'd aim for at least 1 litre of water a day although this will increase in warm weather and when exercising. This is an addition to soup and juice, at least one of which is recommended daily. Many people may also drink a protein shake as well (see Chapter 9).

You may have heard that tea and coffee can lead to dehydration, but the effect they have is mild and caused by caffeine triggering increased urination. The water in caffeinated drinks still counts towards your overall liquid intake and so to some extent one cancels out the other. There is, however, one liquid that does cause dehydration, and has several other effects in the context of GLP, and that's alcohol.

*Alcohol*

In Chapter 3 I touched on how GLP may influence dopamine, the neurotransmitter linked to pleasure and reward. A small study published in *The Journal of the American Medical Association* in March 2025 suggests that GLP's influence on dopamine can have an effect on alcohol consumption, and in some cases lead to a reduced appetite for alcohol.

But if you're taking GLP-1, drinking alcohol can have other effects on the body too, and you may want to bear these in mind regardless of how much you drink:

1. GLP slows down the speed at which food and drink pass through the digestive system, which allows us to feel fuller for longer. But this also means that the alcohol will be absorbed at a slower pace, resulting in a higher level of alcohol staying in your system for longer. This in turn means that you may feel the worse for wear for longer after drinking.
2. Alcohol may exacerbate side effects such as nausea and dizziness that some people experience when taking GLP. You may want to avoid alcohol in the early stages of taking GLP, especially if you experience other side effects.
3. Like GLP, alcohol can cause dehydration so it is essential to ensure you drink plenty of other liquids daily.
4. Alcohol can reduce levels of glucose in the blood, as the liver is busy processing alcohol

at the expense of making glucose. When combined with the effects of GLP, alcohol can potentially lead to hypoglycaemia, the symptoms of which are dizziness, shakiness, lack of concentration and headaches.
5. There is a risk that excessive alcohol consumption can exacerbate sarcopenia, or muscle loss, which I touched on in Chapter 3 – and this can have serious long-term effects.

If you do choose to drink alcohol while taking GLP medications, try to be modest in your consumption and please be mindful that the alcohol level in your bloodstream may stay elevated for longer.

## Variety

*Why?*
A smaller appetite can mean that one enjoys food less, and I have certainly heard from clients that while they are enjoying not having to battle any cravings, the flip side is that they take less pleasure in eating.

In order to retain enjoyment and make it easier to keep up a good intake of food, I advise clients to mix things up with different flavours and textures. Eating a variety of food helps supply various nutrients, each with a slightly different role, as the spread of nutrients differs between even similar foods. To boost nutrient intake, I also recommend soups and juices, as well as wholefoods, as they are easy to eat and are concentrated sources of nutrients.

These elements combine to deliver good nutrition along with a level of weight loss that offsets the potential unwanted side effects of rapid weight loss usually associated with taking GLP medication. Including all these elements should supply the nutrients all adults need to maintain a healthy body.

The clients I have worked with who follow these simple principles have lost weight, but they have done so while still maintaining nutritional health. They have minimal muscle loss, their skin quality is maintained, and they are able to eat plenty of different foods. One particular client has kindly agreed to let me quote her experience using the plan I set out for her and her husband:

> *I hear about people becoming scrawny with wrinkly skin on their arms and a fallen face, and I am sure a few of my friends are taking the jabs because I see the tell-tale signs. But neither D [her husband] nor I have any of those. We eat, we enjoy what we eat, we take our supplements and pay attention to the hunger cues as you directed. D had to tweak his dose as he was finding it hard to eat much, but once his doctor had reduced the*

*dose to what he was taking earlier on, he eats as I do.*

*I do find that I don't really enjoy cooking like I used to but it's easy to cobble together meals that don't require complicated recipes, so neither of us feel we are missing out.*

*We do our exercises as directed and manage two resistance sessions a week. D plays five-a-side and I play tennis when the weather is good enough so it still feels like fun, and we both enjoy what we do.*

*It's hard to provide a negative but neither of us have had any of the unwelcome side effects we were warned about. We're sure it's because of your guidance, not just before we started but for the last year too.*

Female, 48

# 7

## Your daily menus

In the last chapter we looked at the various elements of what constitutes a healthy and varied diet – and how some of these take on added significance in the light of GLP medication. With this in mind, it's useful to apply some guidelines so that what you eat when taking the medication still promotes good health. Being asked to pay close attention to details such as protein and fibre content may seem a bit tedious, but it's vital to think about these elements in order to get the full benefit of both GLP medication *and* nutrition.

So how do you make sure you're increasing your protein and fibre intake, while still focusing on nutrient-rich foods? Bearing in mind that your appetite is going to be reduced, here's an example of a typical day, allowing for a small portion at each meal:

- **Breakfast** Greek yogurt with blueberries and almonds.
- **Snack** Oatcake with cottage cheese.
- **Lunch** Spinach leaves, avocado, tomato, cucumber, salmon, topped with pumpkin seeds.
- **Snack** Protein shake, dates and nut butter.
- **Dinner** Butternut squash soup with added shredded chicken, egg noodles and courgettes.

Now, let's look at the menu again to get an idea of the top-line macronutrients and nutrients each meal and snack provides, along with the quantities, protein, fibre and calories (I've used the MyFitnessPal app as a resource).

## Breakfast

**Low-fat Greek yogurt** *Protein, calcium, vitamin A*
Amount: 3 tbsp
Calories: 28
Protein: 4.3 g

**Blueberries** *Fibre, vitamins A, C, E and K, carotene, manganese*
Amount: 50 g
Calories: 28
Protein: 0.3 g
Fibre: 1.2 g

**Almonds** *Fibre, protein, calcium, iron*
Amount: 12 almonds
Calories: 80
Protein: 3 g
Fibre: 1.5 g
**TOTAL:** 136 calories, 7.6 g protein, 2.7g fibre

## Snack

**Oatcakes** *Fibre*
Amount: 2 oatcakes
Calories: 110
Fibre: 2.2 g

**Cottage cheese** *Protein, calcium, vitamin B12*
Amount: 50 g
Calories: 49
Protein: 5.5 g
**TOTAL:** 159 calories, 5.5 g protein, 2.2 g fibre

## Lunch

**Spinach leaves** *Fibre, vitamins A, C, K, B6 and folate, iron, calcium, magnesium*
Amount: 2 handfuls
Calories: 10
Protein: 1 g
Fibre: 1 g

**Avocado** *Monounsaturated fat, vitamins C, E, K, variety of B vitamins, fibre, potassium, magnesium*
Amount: 75 g (half a medium avocado)
Calories: 153
Protein: 1.4 g
Fibre: 5 g

**Tomato** *Fibre, vitamins A, C and E, calcium, magnesium, folate*
Amount: 1 medium tomato
Calories: 22
Protein: 1.1 g
Fibre: 1.5 g

**Salmon** *Protein, omega-3 fats, vitamin D and wide range of B vitamins, selenium, iron*
Amount: 1 fillet (approx. 113 g)
Calories: 100
Protein: 19 g

**Pumpkin seeds** *Protein, fibre, zinc, manganese, vitamin E*
Amount: 5 g
Calories: 231
Protein: 1.8 g
Fibre: 0.8 g
**TOTAL:** 516 calories, 24.3 g protein, 8.3 g fibre

## Snack

**Protein shake made with water or any milk** *Protein – if made with milk then calcium, vitamins B12 and D, magnesium and iodine*

One scoop of protein powder usually offers around 25 g of protein and contains around 110 calories. The milk options also offer added protein.
*If made with 200 ml water*
Amount: 30 g
Calories: 112
Protein: 25 g
*If made with 200 ml whole milk*
Calories: 132
Protein: 7 g
*If made with 200 ml skimmed milk*
Calories: 70
Protein: 7 g
*If made with 200 ml unsweetened soy milk*
Calories: 64
Protein: 6 g
**TOTAL:** 80 calories (average), 30 g protein (average)

**Dates** *Fibre, copper, vitamin B6 and magnesium*
Amount: 2 Medjool
Calories: 133
Protein: 0.9 g

Fibre: 3.2 g

**Crunchy peanut butter** *Protein, fibre, vitamin E, niacin, magnesium*
Amount: 1.5 tbsp
Calories: 142.5
Protein: 6 g
Fibre: 2.2 g
**TOTAL:** 228 calories, 6.9 g protein, 5.4 g fibre

## Dinner

**Butternut squash soup** *Vitamins A, C and E, manganese, magnesium*
Amount: 200 ml
Calories: 192
Protein: 7.3 g
Fibre: 6.6 g

**Shredded chicken** *Protein, zinc, selenium and B vitamins*
Amount: 113 g
Calories: 149
Protein: 30 g

**Noodles (egg)** *Fibre, protein*
Amount: 60 g
Calories: 210

Protein: 8 g
Fibre: 2 g

**Courgettes** *Fibre, vitamins A, C and K, folate*
Amount: 1 small
Calories: 22
Protein: 2 g
Fibre: 1.9 g
**TOTAL:** 573 calories, 47.3 g protein, 10.5 g fibre

The portions are modest, but eating small amounts at main meals interspersed with a snack caters for an equally small appetite. Yet these nutrition-dense foods deliver a total of 123.8 g protein and 29.1 g fibre, in 1,689 calories. A woman might want to reduce the portion size, or cut out one date, to get nearer to the 1,300–1,500 calorie mark, but even if you ate exactly these amounts, you'd still lose weight.

A man might add a little more chicken, or increase the amount of pumpkin seeds in the lunchtime salad to get to my suggested 1,800 calories. There are plenty of fruits and vegetables included, which contribute to hydration, along with the 1.5 litres of fluid you should be consuming every day too.

If this seems like a lot of food, then remember that these amounts offer the fuel and nutrients required by an adult. This breakdown allows us to see how this typical daily menu delivers on all the points that will help promote health and weight loss, as part of my GLP plan.

- Protein
- Fibre
- Hydration
- Variety
- Calories

## How to build your daily menu

I find that clients adapt to this way of eating in no time. As long as the calorie intake is sufficient to fuel and nourish them, they can adapt the foods to suit them as they wish. They can swap one form of protein for any other, or adjust the menu for a plant-based diet, or a bespoke mixture of proteins and carbohydrates.

Don't feel like a few almonds with your Greek yogurt and berries? Swap them for walnuts, sesame seeds, cashew nuts and so on. If Greek yogurt isn't for you, then have soy or coconut yogurt instead.

Can't eat nuts, or prefer not to? Then find any other protein to replace it.

If you want to introduce grains to your Greek yogurt and berries at breakfast, then feel free to add in some oats, or you might want to swap the berries for a plum.

It's really up to you how you choose to customise each dish, as long as you're sticking to a mixture of proteins and carbohydrates.

When I work with younger clients in a family setting or in schools, it can be fun to encourage them to eat foods from the different food groups by asking them to imagine a fruit machine. I think it's a useful exercise in this context too.

Picture a fruit machine with a lever on one side. You may be familiar with how fruit machines look – the dials inside the little windows spin when you pull the lever, stopping to show an image or icon.

In my version, there are three dials – one each for protein, fruit/vegetables and a grain/complex carb. You can eat anything you want from each food group. That might be a traditional and familiar dish, such as porridge with almonds and apple, but if you like your oats with a slice of beef and some pineapple, go for it. As long as the food group makes an appearance you can combine them in any way you want.

To make this easier, I have come up with the following lists of suggested proteins, both animal- and plant-based. I have included the amount of protein per 100 g to help you out, but that doesn't mean you should only favour those that offer the most protein: the numbers are just a guide.

First, the animal-sourced ones, listed in descending order.

## Meat

| Protein | Per 100 g (cooked) |
|---|---|
| Chicken breast | 31 g |
| Turkey breast | 29 g |
| Rabbit | 27 g |
| Pork tenderloin | 25 g |
| Duck breast (no skin) | 23 g |
| Goat | 23 g |
| Lamb saddle | 23 g |
| Chicken thigh (no skin) | 22 g |
| Cornish hen | 22 g |
| Pork chop | 22 g |
| Pheasant | 21 g |
| Quail | 21 g |
| Veal | 21 g |
| Venison | 21 g |
| Sirloin steak | 24 g |
| Calves' liver | 20 g |
| Turkey thigh | 20 g |
| Chicken liver | 19 g |
| Guinea fowl | 19 g |
| Wild boar | 19 g |

## Fish and seafood

| Protein | Per 100 g (cooked) |
|---|---|
| Tuna | 30 g |
| Octopus | 29.8 g |
| Anchovies | 29 g |
| Herring | 25 g |
| Salmon | 25 g |
| Sardines | 25 g |
| Mackerel | 24 g |
| Mussels | 24 g |
| Prawn (shrimp) | 24 g |
| Halibut | 23.5 g |
| Eel | 23 g |
| Haddock | 23 g |
| Lobster | 20.5 g |
| Cod | 22 g |
| Crab | 19 g |

## Plant-based proteins

| Protein | Per 100 g (cooked) |
|---|---|
| Spirulina | 57 g |
| Tempeh | 19 g |
| Seitan | 19 g |
| Soybeans | 16.6 g |
| Edamame | 11 g |
| Tofu (firm) | 10 g |
| Black beans | 9 g |
| Chickpeas | 9 g |
| Lentils | 9 g |
| Pinto beans | 9 g |
| Kidney beans | 8.7 g |
| Butter beans | 8 g |
| Mung beans | 7 g |
| Peas | 5 g |
| Quinoa | 4.4 g |
| Chia seeds | 4 g |
| Amaranth | 3.8 g |
| Basmati rice | 3.6 g |
| Brussel sprouts | 3 g |
| Long grain brown rice | 2.6 g |

## Dairy and eggs

| Protein | Per 100 g |
|---|---|
| Parmesan | 35.8 g |
| Grana Padano | 33 g |
| Romano | 31.8 g |
| Gruyère | 29.8 g |
| Emmental | 28.4 g |
| Provolone | 26.2 g |
| Cheddar | 25.4 g |
| Edam | 25 g |
| Gouda | 24.9 g |
| Mozzarella | 22.2 g |
| Goat's cheese | 22 g |
| Eggs | 13 g |
| Duck eggs | 12.8 g |
| Ricotta (low-fat) | 11.4 g |
| Cottage cheese | 11.1 g |
| Greek yogurt (low-fat) | 10.3 g |
| Quark | 8 g |
| Skimmed milk | 3.5 g |
| Buttermilk | 3.3 g |
| Whole milk | 3.2 g |

Note that the calories found in dairy products can be high given the fat content. I suggest opting for low-fat options, not only because of the lower calorie count but also because they contain more protein by weight than the full-fat alternatives. However, if you are struggling to eat enough calories, then the full-fat varieties can be useful. As you aren't eating copious amounts of either, don't be fearful of the regular dairy products made from whole and not skimmed milk.

Of course, these foods don't just contain protein: many are classed as complex carbs and offer fibre too.

## Fibre

Fibre is found in two forms: soluble fibre that dissolves in water to make a gel-like substance, and insoluble, which stays more or less intact in the digestive system. We need both types and they are found in familiar plant foods.

Here are some examples of fibre-rich foods, starting with vegetables – the numbers shown give the amount of fibre per 100g. (Note that avocado is listed in both the vegetable and fruit categories because although many people think of it as a vegetable, it is in fact a member of the fruit family).

## Vegetables

| Fibre | Per 100 g |
|---|---|
| Artichokes | 10.9 g |
| Okra | 5.6 g |
| Brussel sprouts | 3.9 g |
| Acorn squash | 3 g |
| Avocado | 2.9 g |
| Carrots | 2.8 g |
| Lima beans | 2.8 g |
| Peas | 2.8 g |
| Spring greens | 2.8 g |
| Kohlrabi | 2.7 g |
| Lentils | 2.7 g |
| Sweet potato (skin on) | 2.7 g |
| Broccoli | 2.5 g |
| Asparagus | 2.2 g |
| Aubergine | 2 g |
| Beetroot | 2 g |
| Cauliflower | 2 g |
| Potatoes | 2 g |
| Green bean | 1.6 g |
| Squash | 1.6 g |

## Grains

| Fibre | Per 100 g |
|---|---|
| Wheat bran | 42.8 g |
| Barley | 17.3 g |
| Oat bran | 15.4 g |
| Rye flour | 13.6 g |
| Wholewheat flour | 12.2 g |
| Granary bread | 6.9 g |
| Rye bread | 5.8 g |
| Bulgur wheat | 4.5 g |
| Sourdough bread | 4.2 g |
| Wholewheat pasta | 3.9 g |
| Teff | 3.7 g |
| Spelt | 3.8 g |
| Quinoa | 2.8 g |
| White bread | 2.7 g |
| Porridge oats | 2.4 g |
| White pasta | 2 g |
| Brown rice | 1.8 g |
| Polenta | 1.5 g |
| Millet | 1.3 g |
| White rice | 0.4 g |

## Fruit

| Fibre | Per 100 g |
|---|---|
| Passionfruit | 10.4 g |
| Avocado | 6.7 g |
| Raspberries | 6.5 g |
| Guava | 5.4 g |
| Blackberries | 5.3 g |
| Pomegranate | 4 g |
| Persimmon | 3.6 g |
| Pear | 3.1 g |
| Kiwi | 3 g |
| Figs | 2.9 g |
| Banana | 2.6 g |
| Apple | 2.4 g |
| Blueberries | 2.4 g |
| Orange | 2.4 g |
| Cherries | 2.1 g |
| Strawberries | 2 g |
| Papaya | 1.7 g |
| Grapefruit | 1.6 g |
| Mango | 1.6 g |
| Plums | 1.4 g |

Now let's have a look at how this all works in real life. I have put together some suggestions for combining the various foods, which show how easy it is to take in sufficient protein and fibre every day.

The primary effect of GLP is to reduce appetite, so, as I've said before, you may find yourself wanting to eat as little as possible. Think of the client who said that when the medication kicked in she could get away with eating just an apple and a slice of cheese for dinner.

However, although the temptation to minimise mealtimes may be strong, I would urge you to see this as a golden opportunity to focus on the nourishment that food provides – remember, nutrients offer the building blocks to maintain a healthy body. With this in mind, the meal and snack options that follow are light and flavourful, easy to eat and prepare, and provide a wide range of essential nutrients to promote optimum nutrition.

## Breakfasts

- A generous two thirds teacup-sized portion of porridge made with any milk, topped up with walnuts and a few berries (or stir in some crunchy almond butter).
- Smoked salmon on toast.
- A palmful of nuts and an apple, if you're short on time.

- One Weetabix with flaked almonds and apple.
- Pâté/fish paste on toasted brown bread.
- Eggs, two, cooked any way plus a cracker or piece of granary bread and some grilled tomato.
- Leftovers also make a decent breakfast – any meat, fish, poultry along with something grain-based (bread, cracker).

## Mid-morning and afternoon snacks

Even with a modest appetite, having something small to eat between main meals helps keep glucose levels stable, and also contributes to a healthy calorie intake to avoid muscle being broken down.

- Leftovers – if you have, say, salmon, mash up what's left with a little yogurt, add some lemon juice and eat with a small serving of pitta or spread on two oatcakes.
- Apple, pear, or kiwi, etc., with almonds, walnuts, seeds.
- Taramasalata or hummus on oatcakes or Ryvita, or with a carrot dipped in the spread.
- Almond, cashew or peanut butter on a rice cake, rye cracker or half a piece of granary bread or toast.
- Chickpeas or any beans with dip, hummus

perhaps; add any herb such as basil, or a dash of Tabasco.
- Sliced chicken breast or hard-boiled egg with radishes.
- One third of a medium avocado mashed up with hot sauce, pumpkin seeds and cherry tomatoes.
- Apple or pear with a small piece of Cheddar or Gruyère cheese.
- One plum with four walnuts.
- Cottage cheese on corn cake.
- A slice of leftover steak with five cherry tomatoes.
- Mixed seeds and a small banana.
- Half a teacup of cooked chickpeas with a teaspoon of Greek yogurt, seasoned.
- One tablespoon of plain yogurt with blackberries.
- Two slices of tempeh wrapped in lettuce leaves.
- A slice of ham or smoked salmon with Cos lettuce on an oatcake.
- Feta cheese with celery crudités.
- A tablespoon of salmon pâté with sesame seeds and cucumber.
- Boiled egg and mushrooms.
- Sauerkraut on a cracker.
- One tablespoon of cubed feta with diced radish.

- A sardine mashed onto two oatcakes.
- Red pepper hummus with raw cauliflower crudités.
- Watermelon with mixed seeds.
- Two teaspoons of avocado sprinkled with sunflower seeds.
- Pickled herring on an oatcake.
- Chicory leaves and a matchbox-sized block of Gouda.

## Main meals

- Grilled steak with green beans, broccoli, courgettes and a generous tablespoon of brown rice or quinoa.
- Vegetable or chicken soup with added shredded chicken, or added chickpeas/lentils/mixed beans.
- Roast lamb with broccoli, peas and a couple of new potatoes.
- Hummus, with tomato, radish, celery, salad leaves; crumble an oatcake and a few sesame seeds over the salad.
- Fish salad topped with pine nuts and some cooked quinoa or brown rice or a piece of toast.
- Grilled fish with two or three green vegetables,

or stir-fry, plus a few new potatoes, rice or quinoa.
- Prawn curry with a lentil dish and a little basmati rice.
- Two hard-boiled eggs, mashed up with a small teaspoon of Greek yogurt, half a diced red pepper and a pinch of curry powder, turmeric, black pepper and sea salt. Serve with salad leaves or spread on oatcakes or toast.
- Boil brown rice or quinoa in chicken or vegetable stock (simply add a stock cube to the water), allow to cool a little, place two tablespoons of the cooked rice on a plate, add a whole small can of sardines, tuna or salmon, then some radishes or celery for crunch.
- Half a medium-sized avocado, tomato, mozzarella and a handful of spinach leaves. Dress with two tablespoons of olive oil mixed with a drizzle of balsamic vinegar.
- Half a medium-sized avocado mashed with dried chilli flakes and sea salt, spread on a small piece of toast.
- Leftover (cold) green beans with crumbled feta cheese and salad leaves.
- Baked halloumi cheese served with sliced beetroot, lettuce and a dressing of horseradish sauce mixed with lemon juice and a little olive oil.

- Sliced leftover chicken served with diced spring onions, Cos lettuce and two crumbled oatcakes.
- Cold Brussels sprouts mixed with two tablespoons of cooked and cooled quinoa (cook in stock) with a matchbox-sized portion of Parmesan cheese grated on top.
- Baked potato with a third of the centre removed and replaced with baked beans. Top with a small amount of grated Cheddar cheese if desired.
- A slice of ham with a baked sweet potato, drizzled with walnut oil and topped with a large pinch of sunflower seeds.
- Two slices of smoked salmon served with a quarter of a medium avocado, lettuce and a slice of granary bread.
- Mixed-bean salad with tahini on oatcakes.
- Ham and vegetable omelette.
- If you prefer a sandwich, use one slice of bread rather than two to account for a smaller appetite. Then choose any protein source you like (meat, fish, tofu, beans, etc.) but remember to add some vegetables, such as tomato, lettuce or peppers.

So, have *any* protein with *any* complex carb – if you want muesli on sliced beef, then go for it, or porridge with hummus, again, that works.

My clients report that eating this way helps them feel energised and satiated, as modest amounts of food in the day creates a slow but steady supply of glucose and energy.

# 8

# Supplements

The world of vitamin, mineral and other supplements can be bewildering. Not only are there multiple brands and blends to choose from but making a choice about what to take is further complicated by clever marketing, with promises of the 'best' sleep, more energy, sharper focus and improved stamina.

Supplements are often considered part of a healthy lifestyle, and their allure is partially based on their aura of being 'natural'. Back in the day I fell for all the marketing and had a shelf in the kitchen that was crowded with tubs and bottles. I am much more organised now and take just a few supplements, but I'm often astonished at the marketing and promotion I see for supplements, mostly on Instagram and other social media platforms. Despite legislation that governs claims about what vitamins and minerals and the like can do for our health, some supplement brands carry on regardless and make bold assertions about their products.

I worry that we end up taking multiple supplements in the hope that they will do 'something', even if we are not quite sure what that 'something' is. Many blends often contain identical nutrients to other products, so we double up, with almost no benefit – and with the potential for some detriment to our health.

Another complexity is that when a nutrient is reproduced and presented in pill or capsule form in a bottle, it seems to take on an identity almost unrelated to the same nutrient when it is sitting on your plate as part of a meal.

Food occupies a different place in our minds and is rarely presented or marketed with reference to specific nutrients. We don't read the words 'energy' or 'immunity' on a pack of, say, brown rice, even though the nutrients found in the rice support both the creation of energy and the immune system.

But if the same nutrients are isolated and replicated and then popped into a bottle, it is commonplace for them to be marketed highlighting what they can do for you. Take a look in any health store and you'll see the supplements on shelves bunched together by function, be that focus, digestion, hair and nails, skin, energy ... And who doesn't want great energy and digestion and ... well ... great *everything*?

To my mind, when thinking about diet and nutrients, it's always food first, supplements second. But in the context of GLP, it's a bit more nuanced.

If you think back to the outline of what constitutes a balanced diet given in Chapter 7, you will see that your meals should be providing you with a full range of nutrients. For example, if we eat at least five generous portions of fruit and vegetables a day, we will benefit from the vitamins they contain (e.g. vitamins A, C, E, K etc.). Similarly, if we ensure that we get at least 25 g or more of fibre a day, then we will enjoy nutrients such as multiple B vitamins and minerals as well.

This is all within the recommended 2,000 or 2,500 calories per day, and although the guidelines may seem a little generalised – as is inevitable for advice that covers a diverse population – they do deliver what we need.

But we know that life is different with GLP medication, as our calorie intake will be lower – how much lower depends on many things, such as health, age, activity levels and dosage. As I outlined in Chapter 7, I do not recommend drastically lowering calorie intake, to avoid the risk of muscle breakdown. Getting the full complement of macronutrients and nutrients in a limited amount of food is also less likely.

Ideally those nutrients will come from food, and so I urge you once again not to undereat – but to focus on nutrient-dense foods whenever you eat. However, this is a handbook for the real world, and so the supplements I recommend will go some way to replace the nutrients that would normally come from food.

## The supplements to take with GLP

Whenever I am asked which supplement to take for a condition, I always check to make sure that my client isn't taking the nutrient or nutrients already. Nutrients are not benign, and they work synergistically, with a complicated interplay. If there's too much of one, levels of another may be suppressed, and there may also be unwanted side effects.

For example, I might suggest a client consider zinc if they have a poor immune system, but ideally they would stick to roughly a 10 mg supplement, and not exceed 25 mg at most, from all sources. This advice also considers the zinc they are likely to be getting from their diet which will also contribute to the upper limit of 25 mg. Excess zinc can suppress copper levels, which is required for energy production and immune system support. Excess zinc can also lead to diarrhoea, which can affect healthy gut bacteria and hydration. So just saying 'Take zinc' isn't a responsible or measured response.

Few clinical studies have explored potential deficiencies linked to specifically to GLP, but there is some evidence to suggest insufficient levels of several macronutrients and nutrients, namely fibre, calcium, iron, magnesium, potassium, choline and vitamins A, C, D, E and K. Interestingly the same research highlighted a potential oversupply of fat as a percentage of total calories consumed, which included both saturated fat and omega-3, together with sodium, riboflavin, niacin and vitamin B12.

Most strikingly, one study from early 2025 stated that some 57 per cent of participants were not even getting 1.2 g of protein per kilo of body weight when taking GLP medication, which is worryingly low when considering the probable muscle loss.

By way of a reminder, you should already be taking a vitamin D supplement, at least 400 IU a day, and anything up to 2,000 IU daily is fine. Most vitamin D supplements contain D3, which is derived from sheep's lanolin, but if you prefer a plant-based version then D2, sourced from algae, is a good alternative.

## What to take

If you are already taking supplements under the advice of a medical and nutrition professional then it is essential you don't take nutrients in supplement form to excess. I urge you to return to your advisor if you are taking GLP, to discuss your individual requirements as the medication is likely to change the situation.

So, what do you take to supplement the nutrients that may be reduced when eating less, plus compensating for the effects of potential muscle loss and associated skin issues? There are many variables here, such as how good your diet is, any medication you might be taking, your age and general health. Assuming you have followed the guidelines given in earlier chapters, here is what will work best for the most of us.

## A multi-nutrient

Multivitamins offer a moderate amount of a wide range of the nutrients found in food and so, in the context of eating less when taking a GLP, it is prudent to top up as many nutrients as possible in the simplest and most convenient way.

There are countless to choose from, ranging from the value supermarket versions to the more costly brands. You do not have to spend large amounts of money or sign up to a monthly supplement subscription (these are overhyped anyway), and I suggest that a mid-range multi will suffice. It doesn't need to contain protein (see below).

You can choose between a tablet or capsule, which often contain a combination of synthetic versions of nutrients, which are quite safe and have been in use for decades. You might also consider a powdered blend, many of which are green in colour and made from ground and dried vegetables, fruit and other plant-based foods, thereby going some way to replicate the nutrients that one would enjoy from a very good diet. As the nutrients are powdered and mixed with water or juice, they tend to be more easily absorbed.

The nutrients that support every function will be represented here, including those that help skin quality, such as vitamins A, C and E, as well as the minerals zinc and selenium.

The advantage of a powdered supplement is that it can be easily combined with a protein supplement, again in powdered form, and mixed with a liquid.

## Protein

As you know full well by now, you really don't want to lose muscle, and so adding some extra protein by way of a supplement is a smart move. But bear in mind that adding in protein doesn't build muscle without taking up the right exercise (see Chapter 9).

You may already to getting protein from your diet, but in case there are days when you don't get enough, taking extra is a simple way to meet requirements. Making a shake combining a multi-nutrient with protein provides a safety net and is easy to drink. There are many different types of supplementary protein to choose from, such as soy, whey, hemp, pea and others, so get one that suits your needs. Whey protein is made from dairy, so choose one of the others if you are following a plant-based diet.

In terms of which is best, the benefit of getting additional protein outweighs any minor differences between the sources of protein. Most packs of protein powder include a scoop to help measure out a standard dose, usually 20–25 g. If you are confident that you eat plenty of protein and include the types of exercise covered in the next chapter, then feel free to have a half dose, or have one every other day. That said, taking the full amount does ensure that protein goals are met (and there's no real downside).

Supplements are there to top up levels of nutrients, not replace them, and a protein one is recommended to make up any shortfall. The protein supplements are added to either water, milk or plant milk to make a shake, which is easy to drink: and while it is satisfying and tasty, it isn't filling and so won't affect your appetite.

In general, I advise clients taking GLP to have one shake mid-morning or afternoon, in addition to a snack. Your snack might be a couple of walnuts, but you'll find plenty of options in my snack list in Chapter 7.

Some clients choose bone broth, rather than a powdered protein supplement, which contains some 16 g per serving protein on average. It can be made at home by adding some animal bones to a pot of water with herbs and simmering for at least twelve hours. Homemade broth is cheaper than buying it in a carton, and also offers collagen.

For what it's worth, I have 25 g of additional protein several times a week. I've opted for a blend of soy, hemp, brown rice, pumpkin and pea proteins, to which I add water and ice, before giving it a good shake. I sometimes add one third of a teaspoon of cocoa powder for flavour, or a quarter teaspoon of matcha powder, or a shot of coffee for a caffeine boost.

## Fibre

As you will have seen in Chapter 4, fibre is an essential part of any diet, and for the most part, we don't get enough, even without the effects of GLP.

Adding extra fibre to the mix of a powdered multi-nutrient and protein is a convenient way to fulfil your nutritional needs, and there are a couple of ways you might do this:

1. **Add fruit and seeds to your shake and blend**
   You can add berries, or some banana – any fruit will do, as will oats, or any nuts or seeds. A small banana, half an apple and 2.5 g of oats will add 7 g of fibre to your total daily intake.

   This mix does require a blender and so won't be practical if you are away from home during the day, although you could prepare it in advance and take it with you if you have access to a fridge. If you add fruit and seeds, the shake makes an ideal alternative to a snack between meals.

2. **Collagen powder** Collagen is a key protein in the body and contributes to the structure of tissue, including tendons, cartilage, bone and skin. Collagen levels reduce with age and its supplementation has long been associated with maintaining skin quality, hence its potential for use during weight loss. Collagen supplements may help skin suppleness and reduce the slackness associated with weight loss, and so takes on an added relevance in the context of GLP.

The effects of collagen supplements are not as clear cut as many of the brands that sell it would have you think. While there are studies available that for the large part show improved hydration and elasticity, most of the studies are funded by the wellness industry. This doesn't automatically discredit the results, but what does undermine the general results is the inconsistency between types of collagen and dosage. We can't say for sure that taking, say, marine collagen at X dose gives better results that a bovine version at another dose. So if you do choose to take collagen then find a brand that you can afford to take consistently and that suits your taste and budget.

Collagen requires vitamin C for absorption and to promote its activity, hence its inclusion in many collagen blends. If it's not there then you can simply take 250 mg in tablet form or add some powder to your shake before mixing it up. You can also add collagen powder to the protein mix as that will have vitamin C in it and saves you taking it later in the day.

One thing to note is that collagen supplements are expensive, and can feel like a sizeable cost if you're already paying for GLP treatment. It's also not easy to quantify the effects of a collagen supplement, as you can't easily compare your own skin quality with or without a collagen supplement when taking a GLP.

With this in mind, if you do choose to take a collagen supplement, then simply having it every other day should still provide benefits but at half the cost. Whether you feel collagen is worth the investment is ultimately your decision, but if it doesn't break the bank then it can be a useful addition.

3. **Omega-3** Omega-3 fats play many roles, ranging from offsetting inflammation to reducing the risk of cardiovascular disease. They also help skin integrity and hydration. Omega-3 fats

are found in food, namely oily fish, walnuts and chia seeds, amongst others.

There is a case for taking omega-3 fats as a supplement in the context of GLP, but they cannot be taken if you are on medication for blood pressure. Equally, if you are taking aspirin then omega-3 may not be for you, as both can thin the blood and in excess this can increase the potential for poor wound healing and bleeds.

On average, 1000 mg omega-3 a day will suffice. If you eat oily fish then you can take a supplement on days that you aren't eating fish – there's no need to double up.

# 9

# The importance of exercise

*I never liked sport, and the thought of going to a gym used to terrify me because I was so unfit and heavy that I knew people would be staring at me.*

*Once I lost weight it just felt like I wouldn't need to exercise, which at first was a relief. It took me a while to acknowledge that, yes, I was slimmer, but I had no tone at all. I still can't face a gym, but I found some classes which I did online, and while I didn't think it helped much at first, I stuck with it and it's been great.*

*Exercise was only ever something I did because I had to, that's what I felt, but it wasn't until I properly understood the link between what I ate, and not just how much I ate, that I really saw the changes. I now eat more protein and – combined with the online classes – I can really see a difference in my tone and how I look.*

*Now that it feels like a choice and not a chore, I really enjoy it – and have way more energy, too.*

Female, 41

*It was always the same. I'd start a diet and force myself to go to the gym, I even got a trainer one year as I thought that paying all that money would make me go more often.*

*When I started and then stopped my medication the first time I didn't bother with the gym as despite the awful side effects, mostly nausea and dizziness, I lost 6 kg, so I felt like I didn't need to make the effort. It wasn't until I switched meds and got the dose right that I started exercising again.*

*I had experienced wasting muscles at first, but when I restarted the jabs I felt motivated. I got some resistance bands and watched classes online, starting gently at first. I can't claim to enjoy it much, but I do it because I know I need to, and I can't be spending all this money on the injections without putting in the extra effort.*

Male, 48

When it comes to weight management, diet and exercise are two sides of the same coin. It is clear that in order to lose weight you need to eat less and move more. If you have any doubts about that, think of the way diets are promoted in January (after the Christmas break), and how gym membership and attendance shoot up at the same time.

I worked with a group of personal trainers for a while and when I asked them about the most common reason for members to join the gym, they all said, in unison, 'Lose weight and tone up'. But exercise is good for all of us – whether or not we are taking GLP – and the benefits go far beyond just burning calories. If one of the main reasons you might have exercised in the past was to lose weight, then it's possible that you may not feel motivated to exercise when taking GLP medication, as the benefits will be less obvious at first. But, as we will see in this chapter, exercise takes on special relevance in this situation. As we know, a cut in calories results in an energy deficit, and so energy stored in fat cells has to be released. This gap can be maximised by increasing energy requirements through physical activity.

## Benefits of exercise

Being active and exercising are two different things, and both have wide-ranging benefits.

1. **Weight and muscle mass** Combining cardio – be that walking, cycling or running – with resistance training will go some way to preserving lean muscle. Muscles are also more efficient at using energy as they are more active than inactive fat cells. Therefore, having more muscle means that the body will be more metabolically active, in other words use more energy. Consistent exercise also improves insulin sensitivity and reduces abdominal fat, both of which are linked to a lower risk of disease.
2. **Bone density** Weight-bearing and resistance exercises are essential for maintaining strong, healthy bones. Activities like walking, running and lifting weights stress the bones just enough to trigger new bone growth. This is particularly important as we age, since bone density naturally declines, increasing the risk of fractures and osteoporosis. Resistance training has been shown to increase bone-mineral density, especially in post-menopausal women and older adults.

    For more information on the nutrients that assist in maintaining bone density see Chapter 4.
3. **Longevity** Physical activity reduces the risk of chronic illnesses such as heart disease, cancer and type 2 diabetes in various ways. Exercise

helps regulate blood pressure, can improve cholesterol and other lipids in the blood profiles and boosts immune function (but overtraining does the opposite, hence the need for moderation).

Even moderate activity, such as brisk walking for thirty minutes a day, has been shown to lower mortality risk.

4. **Brain health** Exercise has profound benefits for brain health, affecting cognitive function and also potentially helping to alleviate low mood and depression.

Physical activity increases blood flow to the brain, delivering oxygen and nutrients that support its normal function. Regular exercise has been shown to support the formation of new neurons, a process called neurogenesis, notably in the hippocampus part of the brain, which is key for learning and memory.

Regular activity reduces stress, anxiety and depression by balancing neurotransmitters like serotonin and dopamine.

## Muscle mass, protein and exercise

In the context of GLP, muscle loss happens because of eating too little, and from not ensuring decent amounts of protein in the diet. But we can't just eat protein and expect it to miraculously end up as muscle mass. The amino acids that are contained in protein need to have a reason to be directed to the muscles rather than anywhere else in the body, and that is done by challenging or stressing the muscle so that it requires repairs.

When we exercise – and this happens when we're engaging in any sort of weight-bearing activity – we actually cause tiny tears in our muscles. So, if you imagine lifting a weight to strengthen the biceps in your arms, that extra weight stresses the muscle and that's what causes these small tears that are, effectively, damage.

As you may remember from Chapter 4, protein consists of amino acids, which are the raw materials the body uses to build and repair tissue. Amino acids are used to repair the tears, adding to the muscle mass in a process called muscle protein synthesis.

So, one side of the equation is supplying the amino acids from our diet; the other is creating the 'draw' for them to be sent to the muscles to repair the tears.

Protein and amino acids are used all over the body, so in order to ensure that the muscle mass is maintained there has to be a surplus of both. This is why maintaining a diet with sufficient protein is vital, especially when you're eating less on GLP. As mentioned in the previous chapter, a protein supplement is a good way to ensure that you're meeting your protein needs (although what you eat is important as well).

If you consistently consume enough protein, especially after workouts, your body can maintain muscle mass rather than use it as a source of fuel. But this *only* works if the muscles have been challenged thereby effectively attracting amino acids so that they might be used for repair and maintenance.

Without the right type of exercise, eating additional protein is simply just calories. Eating extra chicken or fish or tofu isn't enough. We have to do our bit too ... and that's where exercise comes in.

## Which exercise?

Both cardiovascular and weight-bearing exercise have benefits, whether or not you're taking GLP medication.

Historically, the way that men and women feel about weight training can be quite different. This isn't the place for a deep dive into muscles, gender and aesthetics, but I have heard countless times over the years that some women are concerned about using weights as they worry about getting 'muscly'.

That could be a legitimate concern if one was eating, say, 3,000 calories a day with many grams of protein and doing some serious weight training too. The same would be true for either sex, but unless that's what you are aiming for, the sort of weight-bearing exercise you should do is much more moderate.

I am not an expert in this field, but I am very pleased that Joe Warner, the former editorial director of *Men's Fitness* magazine and one of the UK's most high-profile fitness journalists, has agreed to offer his expert advice.

I asked Joe to choose some important exercises that engage and maintain muscles. If you have any concerns about these or similar exercises, then please speak with an appropriate professional.

## Squats

*What*
The number one lower-body lift that works your legs, bum and core. No kit needed – your own body weight is enough at first.

*Why*
Squats power everyday movement: getting out of a chair, getting up off the loo, picking things up. They're also a compound, multi-joint movement, meaning that they work several major muscle groups at the same time – making them one of the most effective exercises for building and maintaining muscle mass and strength. Stronger legs mean stronger bones, better balance, fewer aches and injuries, and they make life easier – from daily chores to a game of tennis.

*How*
Stand tall with your feet shoulder-width apart. Tense your tummy by pretending someone's about to poke your belly button. With your arms straight out in front of you or down by your sides, push your hips back, bend your knees, and lower your bum down as if you're sitting down. Go as low as feels comfortable – aim for thighs parallel to the floor – then push through your heels to stand back up. That's one rep. Do two or three sets of 10–15 reps, resting for a couple of minutes between sets.

*Next steps*
When you're ready, you can make the move tougher by slowing down the lowering phase or adding a brief pause in the bottom position. Or you can add extra weight: hold a dumb-bell in each hand by your sides, or grip a kettlebell in both hands at chest height (called a goblet squat).

## Lunges

*What*
Another classic lower body move that also works your legs, bum and core, while improving your balance and coordination.

*Why*
Lunges are a compound move like squats because they work multiple muscles at once, and because they're a single-leg exercise, they build strength and muscle mass equally across both legs. They're also a functional movement with huge crossover benefit to everyday life – think climbing the stairs, walking uphill or getting up from the floor.

*How*
Stand tall with your feet hip-width apart and hands on your hips. Take a big step forward with your left leg, then bend both knees to lower down until your left thigh is parallel to the floor and your right knee is just above the ground. Keep your torso upright and your left knee over your left ankle. Push through your left foot to return to the start. That's one rep. Do 8–12 reps leading with your left leg, then do the same, leading with your right leg. That's one set. Do two or three sets, resting for a couple of minutes between sets.

*Next steps*
Make body-weight lunges more challenging by slowing down each rep or pausing for a second at the bottom position. You can also try variations like reverse lunges (step back instead of forward), walking lunges (taking continuous steps forward with each lunge) or lateral lunges (step to the side). You can also hold a

dumb-bell in each hand to increase the workload on your muscles.

## Deadlifts

*What*

A multi-muscle move that works your back, legs, bum and core in one powerful lift. It's best done with some extra resistance, like a kettlebell or a pair of dumb-bells.

*Why*

Deadlifts strengthen the entire back of your body – what trainers call the 'posterior chain' – so they're a great antidote to long days spent sitting down. They mimic the simple act of picking something up from the floor and protect your lower back by teaching you to lift properly using your legs and hips, not by rounding your spine. In short, they're one of the top moves for building muscle and strengthening bones.

*How*

Stand tall with your feet hip-width apart, in front of a pair of dumb-bells or a kettlebell. Keeping your back flat, bend your knees to lower down, then take hold of a dumb-bell in each hand, or the kettlebell in both hands. With your back straight and core braced, push through your heels and squeeze your bum to stand up, lifting the weight straight up. Pause at the top, then lower back down under control to return the weight to the floor. Let go and stand back up. That's one rep. Do two or three sets of 10–15 reps, with a couple of minutes' rest between sets.

*Next steps*
Once you've mastered the movement, you can gradually increase the weight you lift, using dumb-bells, kettlebells or a barbell. Or try variations: Romanian deadlifts (RDLs) keep your legs straighter, so work your hamstrings and lower back more, and you don't put the weight down between reps, so your muscles work much harder for faster size and strength gains.

## Step-ups

*What*
A smart and simple move that works your legs, bum and core. All you need is a sturdy step, box or bench – around knee height is ideal.

*Why*
Step-ups are another functional move that mimic the real-life movements your body was built for. As well as strengthening all your major lower-body muscles, they also boost balance, coordination and concentration, and support stronger bones, healthier joints and more

resilient connective tissue – helping you stay active and injury free.

*How*

Stand tall in front of your step or box. Put your left foot on top, keeping your chest up and back straight, then push through that foot to lift your body up, so your right foot is on the box too. Step back down, left foot first. That's one rep. Do 10–15 reps leading with your left leg, then switch legs. That's one set. Do two or three sets, resting for a couple of minutes between sets.

*Next steps*

To make the move harder, adjust the height of the box or use extra weight, like a dumb-bell in each hand or a kettlebell in both hands held against your chest. For a more explosive exercise to fire up your muscles, do box jumps: stand in front of the box, then jump with both feet to land on top of it, before stepping back down to repeat.

## Push-ups

*What*

Also known as press-ups, this is the one exercise everybody knows – it's the go-to move in films and fitness tests to prove how athletic someone is. A compound lift that works your chest, shoulders, arms and core all at once, it only requires your body weight, a little space and some effort.

*Why*
Push-ups build and maintain upper-body muscle, improve joint stability in your shoulders and elbows, and strengthen your core. They're also one of the only moves that work your chest and shoulders without requiring specialist kit and have a knock-on benefit for real life – like pushing open heavy doors or getting up from the floor.

*How*
Start on the floor with your arms straight, hands shoulder-width apart, and on your toes so your body forms a straight line from head to heels. Brace your core, then bend your elbows to lower your chest towards the floor. Stop just before it makes contact, then push through your hands to return to the start. That's one rep. Do 5–10 reps per set, and aim for two or three sets, resting for a couple of minutes between sets.

*Next steps*
If full push-ups feel too tough, you've got options. Either start with your knees on the floor, or elevate your hands on a step or bench. To make them harder, slow down the movement, add a pause at the bottom, or move your hands closer together.

## Overhead press

*What*

A compound upper-body exercise that works your shoulders, upper chest, arms and core. You'll need some dumb-bells or a resistance band – as well as a high ceiling.

*Why*

The overhead press builds muscle mass and strength where many people lose it as they age – the shoulders, chest and arms – and works the rotator cuff, a collection of small but important stabilising muscles responsible for shoulder joint health and mobility. It's also highly functional – mimicking daily movements like lifting bags, stacking boxes or reaching high shelves.

*How*

Stand tall with your feet hip-width apart, holding a dumb-bell in each hand at shoulder height with palms facing forward. Brace your core and bum, then press the weights directly up until your arms are straight and the weights are overhead. Pause, then lower with control back to the start. That's one rep. Aim for 8–12 reps per set, and do two or three sets with a couple of minutes' rest between sets.

*Next steps*
To make the move more challenging, do the move seated (which takes your legs out of the equation), try single-arm presses (which test your balance and core), or use heavier dumb-bells. Whichever version you do, keep each rep smooth and controlled to build strength without risking injury.

## Bent-over row

*What*
An unrivalled upper body move to strengthen your upper and lower back, arms and core. You'll need a pair of dumb-bells or a kettlebell.

*Why*
Bent-over rows build muscle across your back, shoulders and arms to improve strength, power and posture. They also train the smaller muscles that support your spine and shoulder joints – reducing the risk of injury – and make many everyday tasks, like carrying groceries, lifting luggage or picking up kids, much easier.

*How*
Stand tall with a dumb-bell in each hand. Keeping your back flat, knees soft and core braced, hinge at the hips so your torso is leaning forward at around a 45-degree angle. Let the weights hang below your shoulders

with straight arms. This is the start position. Row the weights up to your torso by bending your elbows and squeezing your shoulder blades together. Pause at the top, then lower with control. That's one rep. Do 8–12 reps per set, and aim for two or three sets with a couple of minutes' rest between sets.

*Next steps*
Make the move easier by doing single-arm rows with a light weight and one knee and hand supported on a bench. Make it harder with heavier weights, slower reps, or a longer pause and hold in the top position. Just always ensure your back is straight and each rep is controlled: rounding your back, twisting your torso or yanking the weight up is asking for trouble.

Joe's advice is great, but you may also want to consider working with a personal trainer. I have clients who have paid for a few sessions with a trainer and then carried on at home with online classes – you can find free options on YouTube. Other clients have been training for years, and focus more on resistance training while still including cardio work, albeit a little less.

You may prefer sport to a gym, or group fitness classes, or boxing or Pilates ... there's a long list. You really must get expert advice from a trainer or fitness professional, and make sure they know you are taking GLP medication and what your goals are.

# 10

# Looking to the future

It is important to be realistic when it comes to 'life after GLP'. When intake of GLP stops, there is every chance that the impaired glucose control will contribute to the amount of weight and speed at which it is regained. There is a suggestion that if muscle mass has reduced as well, then appetite may increase to higher than previous levels, although that's hard to quantify due to the current lack of targeted research.

Cost aside, GLP medication can be considered easier than living with the tyranny of dieting and that repetitive cycle of losing weight and then regaining the same weight – or even more.

## What happens when the medication is stopped?

In Chapter 1, we looked at how the medications work by mimicking the effects of two hormones that are produced naturally in the human body.

Collectively, they combine to improve glucose management and slow digestion resulting in a smaller appetite and so, in the real world, we eat less, and weight loss follows. But what if the medication is stopped? The consequences are obvious – and unfortunate.

The influence of the medication wears off, appetite returns, the food noise gets turned up, and, if we eat more, then weight is regained. Some longer-term studies have shown that people who had lost weight with a GLP regained some two-thirds of the weight within twelve months of stopping the medication. Moreover, a systematic review and meta-analysis of data presented at the European Congress on Obesity in 2025 by the Nuffield Department of Primary Health Sciences at Oxford University showed that users can expect to regain all the lost weight within twenty-four months of stopping medication. Matters are complicated because the National Institute for Health and Care Excellence (NICE) recommend that GLP is not taken for more than two years via the NHS, not because it stops working but because of limited space within the specialist services for obesity. This may drive people towards the private sector until such time as the guidelines for prescribing GLP change.

We should understand that obesity is a chronic disease, as recognised by the World Health Organisation in 1997. According to WHO, obesity is a 'serious, chronic, and complex disease, requiring prevention and management strategies at both individual and societal levels'. The risks of obesity and being overweight include an increased likelihood of type 2 diabetes, cardiovascular disease and certain types of cancer.

I am certainly not advising you or anyone else to stay on the medication for life, or indeed to stop taking it. The decision to do so is personal, and involves several factors that are down to each of us.

## Dose management

The advice given here is based largely on my experience of working with clients who have been, or are taking, GLP-1 medication.

Remember that the drugs were initially developed and thus licensed to help patients living with type 2 diabetes, and any ensuing weight loss was considered a side effect. Prescribing them for weight loss was considered to be 'off label', although more recently the weight-loss effects have been licensed too.

Therefore, my question is this: if there is an ideal dose, one that allows you to get to a place where hunger is quite manageable, where you can still look forward to food, to eat and enjoy it but in amounts that help you lose and maintain a weight, without side effects or unwelcome consequences, what reason is there not to continue?

And if there is an optimal dose – which may be different for you than for someone else – which can be identified, is that the ideal outcome?

Although these drugs have been around for many years, well before their weight-loss potential dominated the news, we don't as yet know if there might be any unpleasant long-term consequences of prolonged use.

But remember that people managed their weight before the advent of GLP. While the medications do a lot of the heavy lifting for you, they are simply a tool. When working with clients who are managing the transition away from GLP, we look at the way the body makes GLP naturally. Bear in mind that the medication mimics these hormones and that eating triggers GLP production. Therefore, eating little and often, ensuring that meals and snacks contain a combination of protein, carbohydrates and fat, will go some way to offset changes in appetite.

There's more, as the way that the body handles glucose is improved due to reduced fat levels and better insulin sensitivity. Therefore, the reduction in fat that has been achieved during GLP treatment contributes to easier appetite control.

But we must be realistic. I have several clients who have worked with their doctor to reduce or cease GLP medication who then go on to manage their weight. But it's not always easy, and everyone will respond differently to the changes.

## Conclusion

When I first started working with clients taking GLP medications to support the management of type 2 diabetes, it would have been hard to predict that within a decade those same drugs would be adapted and repurposed to offer a solution for obesity and weight loss. The outcome, as we all know, is that highly effective GLP medications can change lives with an ease that was previously unimaginable.

For most people with a high BMI, a 20 per cent decrease in body weight will address health factors that would have resulted in an increased risk of disease. For example, it's likely that blood pressure will be normalised, while raised cholesterol and the level of other fats in the blood will be lowered – leading to a reduced risk of a cardiovascular event. Achieving a healthy BMI can also help improve insulin sensitivity which, as you will know from earlier chapters, can make energy production more efficient.

Weight loss will likely ease joint pain and improve

mobility, while reducing the likelihood of developing some forms of cancer, especially those of the bowel, kidney, liver, breast and uterine cancer.

Achieving a healthy weight has been a battle for millions of people, but GLP medications have offered a solution. Their advent has been remarkable: from the initial innovation that brought them to the market, to the design of the pens, ease of use and availability, it's not hard to understand why they're so popular. And improvements are on the cards too, with the next generation of GLP drugs likely to be available in pill and tablet form, offering an alternative to the jabs.

When the medication is taken wisely and under appropriate supervision, the results can be spectacular. GLP is a potent tool and needs to be handled with care, which includes how we access it, the side effects, dosages and long-term use. This is always best done by working closely with your doctor, specialist or expert pharmacy, and ensuring regular contact and supervision, especially when upping doses – tempting though it may be, I strongly advise against going it alone.

GLP medications are not always plain sailing as they won't suit everyone, and the side effects can range from mild to serious. I cannot stress enough how essential it that you work only with an appropriate health professional and inform them of any and all side effects.

One might consider very rapid weight loss as a welcome outcome, but I consider it to be a worrying side effect. Unless weight loss is modest and managed, there may be real world consequences. As you will have seen in the previous chapters, I believe that eating too little presents a risk – and the more stories I hear, the more concerned I am that the promise of very easy weight loss has eclipsed the threat of the longer-term effects of undereating.

Rapid weight loss has repercussions, which include the all-important loss of muscle (see Chapter 3) and an increased risk of a whole host of nutrient deficiencies (see Chapter 5). It may not be easy to strike a happy balance between reducing your appetite to optimise weight loss and eating enough to support your nutritional requirements. It's a fine line and in my experience requires an awareness of not only how much we are eating but of what we eat when we want to eat less.

When you're using the jab, it's common for the starter dose to be increased after a few weeks or months with increases continuing until you reach the maximum dosage. I can appreciate why this might be attractive for clients, as each increase comes with the promise of greater and easier weight loss and it can be easy to overlook the progress that has already been made. In some cases increases are also normalised by providers, who will email clients when they think it's time to up the dosage.

It sounds innocuous enough, but however you get the medications, my advice is to think hard about where you were, how you eat now, the weight you have lost to date, your skin quality, muscle tone and your goals before automatically increasing the dose. I am not a doctor, but I think that just because you can increase the dose, doesn't mean you have to.

If your current dose allows you to eat less, but to eat well and to avoid the pitfalls of rapid weight loss, then I urge you to speak to a medical professional before making any changes to your dosage. Ask yourself, and them, if you need to increase the dose and if so, why and what you might expect with the next dose.

With all this in mind, let me leave you by wishing you the best of luck with the GLP experience. GLPs are impressive medications, affording the opportunity to achieve a healthier weight. They can offer the chance to reframe what you eat and see food as nourishment, and free yourself from the diet trap. Think of eating well like a nutritional pension, planning ahead for a healthier future.

Please ensure that you eat enough, get the protein and fibre your body needs, do that weight bearing exercise, avoid muscle loss, take the right supplements and do not hurry to increase your dose if it's working for you.

Lastly, I have a clinic in London and see clients in person and online, and I would be very happy if you'd like to get in touch to talk about personal consultations, be that for GLP or any other aspect of nutrition and diet. You can find me at: ianmarber.com

# Acknowledgements

As ever, special thanks Amanda Preston, for all that she and her colleagues do for me. And, of course, to Bernadette Marron and everyone at Piatkus.

I am very grateful to Dr Ellie Cannon for her generous introduction and support, and to Joe Warner for his expert contribution.

With thanks to my old friend Tracy, who called me and told me to write this book.

I am especially indebted to the countless people who were kind enough to share their GLP experiences and stories. I am truly grateful for your time and honesty.

## About the author

**Ian Marber** is a renowned UK nutrition therapist, best-selling author and award-winning health writer. Known for his practical and balanced approach, Ian has advised more than 20,000 private clients at his London clinic.

After graduating in 1999, he founded the nutritional consultancy, The Food Doctor. Since his departure from the consultancy in 2012, Ian has continued to work with individuals and industry professionals alike, leading seminars and workshops, and collaborating with high-profile food and hospitality brands. He is also a regular contributor to print media, TV and radio, and has published fourteen books on nutrition.